CP NOW is a South Carolina non-profit corporation
Post Office Box 8347
Greenville, SC 29604

COVER PHOTO CREDIT

Dandelion by slgckgc
https://www.flickr.com/photos/slgc/8681169825
Note: Text added to cropped original photo

Dear Parents and Family,

The period after you hear about your child or family member's diagnosis feels overwhelming and often scary. This resource has been created with you in mind, by parents of children with CP who have been where you are now, and who want to tell you that **you are not alone**.

You may not know where to begin in the CP Tool Kit or where to find the strength to open the pages before you. **Take your time and know that you do not have to read everything in a day or even a week or even a few months**. Some days you will feel stronger and more prepared to learn than others. The Tool Kit may be used like an encyclopedia, referencing sections as needed, or some of you may find relief by reading it in order from cover to cover. However you decide to approach the Tool Kit, be gentle with yourself and use the information to empower you and your family.

Our cover includes a large picture of a dandelion. Dandelions symbolize positivity, hope and survival, often finding unthinkable ways to emerge through cracks in the sidewalk. I have been fascinated by how the qualities of the dandelion have captured our experience with our daughter whose persistence and resilience have repeatedly surprised us. As we move further from the day when my daughter was diagnosed with cerebral palsy, the playfulness of the dandelion has also been a gentle reminder to simply enjoy each other as mother and daughter, outside of doctor and therapy visits and her diagnosis of cerebral palsy.

I have wanted to pursue this CP Tool Kit project since the day my daughter was diagnosed with cerebral palsy and our family struggled to find the information and support we needed. Our team of passionate and dedicated parents and professionals have worked together to bring you a comprehensive resource about early brain injury/disturbances leading to cerebral palsy. It is our goal to empower you with the knowledge you need to ask important questions, advocate for your child, and strengthen your family.

Sincerely,

Michele Shusterman
Founder and Executive Director of CP NOW

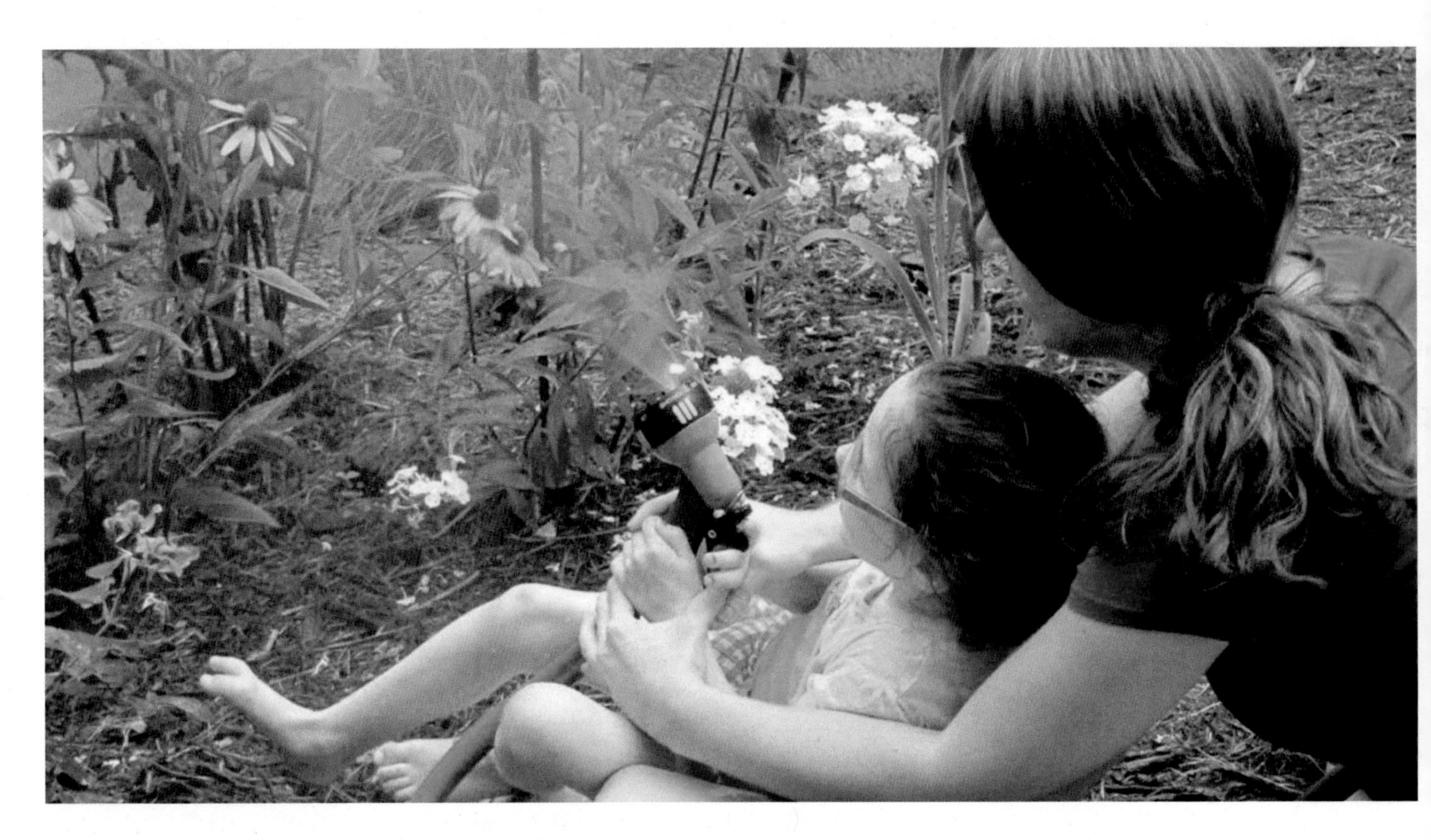

IF YOU ARE READING THIS, someone you love or care for has been diagnosed with cerebral palsy. Cerebral palsy, or "CP" for short, describes a group of movement disorders caused by an injury or disturbance in the early developing brain, and specifically the areas involved with creating movement.

When parents and families get a diagnosis of CP, they often feel confused about what the diagnosis means for their child's future. They wonder what to do to best help their child. Emotional reactions can be strong and decisions can be difficult. **Although the diagnosis of cerebral palsy may feel overwhelming, it does not define or dictate what your loved one's future will look like.** Discoveries in neuroplasticity, and research into the brain's ability to change and recover from injuries like those that cause CP, are offering new insight and hope for the CP community.

The Cerebral Palsy Tool Kit was created to help you sort through some of these emotions and answer your questions and concerns related to CP. It will guide you through the initial diagnosis period, direct you to other helpful resources and provide information to you about the different approaches to treating and managing CP.

The CP Tool Kit Parent Leadership Committee
Jennifer Lyman
Anna Meenan
Lori Poliski
Michele Shusterman
Christina Youngblood

Contents

1 About CP 4
What is it? 4
Co-occurring conditions 5
Is there a cure for CP? 6

2 Data and Statistics 7

3 Diagnosing CP 8
How is CP diagnosed? 8
Types of CP 9
How does a CP diagnosis help your child? 13
Accepting a diagnosis of CP 14

4 Who else has CP? 17

5 After the Diagnosis—Creating Your Child's Team 22
Coordinating care 22
Early assessments and screenings 26

6 You, Your Family and CP 40
Sharing the diagnosis with family and friends 40
Pitfalls of predictions 43
Impact of a CP diagnosis on family 44

7 Early Intervention & Early Education 47
What is early intervention? 47
Daycare and preschool 48

8 Thinking Through Treatments 50
Treating CP is not one size fits all 50
The treatment decision checklist 50

9 Treatments/Interventions Glossary 52
PT, OT and speech 52
Treatments by movement disorder type 55
General orthopedic procedures for CP 59
Complementary or Alternative Medicines (CAMs) 60
Creating a balanced therapy program 62
Assistive Technology (AT) 64
Equipment, durable medical goods and orthoses 64

10 Insurance and Special Needs Planning 66
Health insurance 66
Achieving a Better Life Experience (ABLE) Act 69
Special needs trusts 69

11 Advocacy and Awareness Days 70

12 Supportive Words from Other Parents 71

13 Additional Resources 72
CDC data and statistics 72
Local resources 72
AACPDM Professional Member Directory 72
Assistive Technology 72
General child care resources 72
Insurance/financial planning resources 73
Oral Health 73
Respite care 73
Vision 73
Books 73

14 Contributors 74

15 References 76

16 Glossary 78

SECTION 1

About CP

What is It?

CP IS THE MOST COMMON CAUSE OF motor disability in children and also affects a large adult population.[1] **The term cerebral palsy describes a group of movement disorders caused by an injury or disturbance in the early developing brain and specifically the areas involved with creating, coordinating and controlling movement and posture.** It is generally accepted that in cases where cerebral palsy is diagnosed, interferences in brain development have occurred in the fetal or infant brain before the age of two years. This is in contrast to later brain injuries such as a traumatic brain injury (TBI) where brain development is further along when the injury occurs.

Early interferences in the areas of the brain involved with movement can lead to problems with how the brain communicates with the muscles. It may cause difficulty with some or all of the following motor skills: coordination, muscle tone (too tight or too loose), reflexes, posture and balance. When these problems are identified and persist, and other conditions are ruled out, it is called cerebral palsy. Most people with CP have a typical lifespan. Although cerebral palsy is not progressive, the presentation and symptoms may change over time as the brain develops further and there is ongoing wear and tear on the muscles, tendons, and bones.

Some of the conditions that have been associated with an increased risk for cerebral palsy include infection, infant stroke, multiple births, prematurity, genetics, and other problems related to blood and oxygen moving to and throughout the developing brain. Researchers are looking at what happens under these conditions to cause cerebral palsy and why some of these conditions do not always lead to CP. For instance not all babies born prematurely develop cerebral palsy, but many people who have CP were born prematurely. What makes some premature infants more vulnerable than others? These are the kinds of questions that still need to be answered to help us advance efforts toward prevention and improve treatment.

Individuals who have CP are affected differently depending on where and how the disturbance in brain development occurred. Whereas one person may have trouble with movement on one side of the body including their hand, arm and leg, another may have difficulty sitting up, maintaining balance, and using all four limbs. Since there are muscles throughout the entire body, it's important to keep in mind that in addition to the obvious large muscles and muscle groups that may be affected, even tiny muscles, like, for example, those controlling and coordinating eye movements, may be involved as well.

Parents often become confused about how conditions such as infant stroke, infant asphyxia, static encephalopathy, periventricular leukomalacia (PVL) and others relate to CP. These conditions and others, are events that are part of the umbrella of conditions that may lead to the disturbances in brain development that cause CP. However, once your child has a diagnosis of CP, or other associated conditions (such as epilepsy), they will often replace these terms. This is because the new diagnoses capture the resulting set of persistent symptoms and disorders for which the child will now be treated.

Co-Occuring Conditions/Problems related to CP:

These are not all of the possible conditions seen in people who have CP. Consult with your medical team for further information about your particular concerns and more information.

PAIN

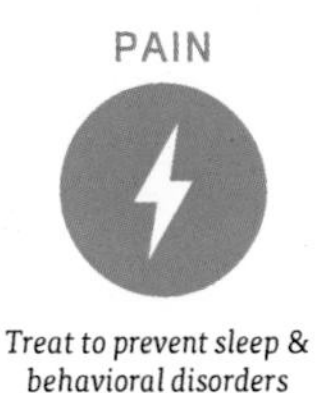

Treat to prevent sleep & behavioral disorders

HIP DISPLACEMENT

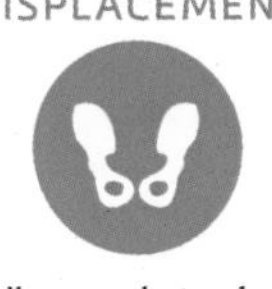

Talk to your doctor about regular monitoring

SCOLIOSIS AND CONTRACTURES

Talk to your doctor about regular monitoring

INTELLECTUAL

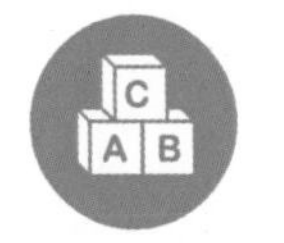

May have more difficulty with academics and social skills

COMMUNICATION

Augment communication early

EPILEPSY

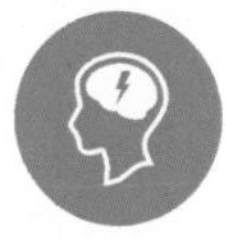

Seizures will resolve for 10–20%

BEHAVIOR DISORDER

Treat early & ensure pain is managed

INCONTINENCE

Investigate source/s of incontinence & allow more time

SLEEP DISORDER

Conduct investigations & ensure pain is managed

VISION

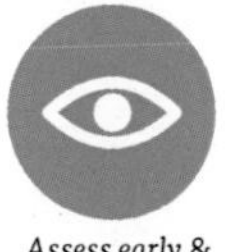

Assess early & accommodate

NON-ORAL FEEDING

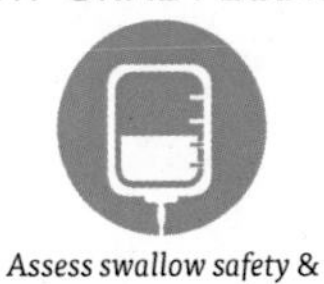

Assess swallow safety & monitor growth

HEARING

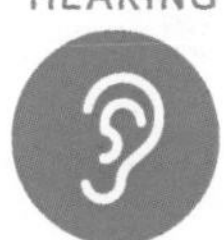

Assess early & accomodate

Adapted in part from the World CP Day Diagnosis and Treatment Infographic, worldcpday.org

Co-Occurring Conditions

Co-occurring conditions are medical conditions that may be seen along with the primary diagnosis of cerebral palsy. Some of these are secondary conditions which develop as a result of having CP. These include things like difficulty swallowing, constipation and problems with hip development or bladder function. Other impairments or disorders called associated conditions, are related to the initial disturbances in brain development which may have affected areas outside of motor function. These may include epilepsy, visual perceptual disorders or disturbances in the onset of puberty. **Please keep in mind that although it is helpful to be aware of these conditions, having cerebral palsy does not automatically mean your child will have all of them.** It is likely however that they will have some of these issues. For this reason it is important to be aware of these conditions so that you can access timely treatment and support whenever possible.

There may be musculoskeletal problems such as:

- → Abnormal hip development and alignment
- → Contractures
- → Scoliosis

Other related conditions may involve problems with:

- → Behavior/Emotional
- → Bladder function
- → Communication and speech
- → Digestion and constipation (which may affect continence)
- → Eating and drinking
- → Early or delayed puberty
- → Epilepsy
- → Hearing
- → Intellectual impairments
- → Learning/processing information
- → Perception
- → Saliva loss/drooling
- → Sensory Integration
- → Sleep disorders
- → Visual impairments

Each child with CP is unique and may present with only a few of these conditions or perhaps several. **Later in the Tool Kit we discuss assessments and screenings for some of these potential problems.**

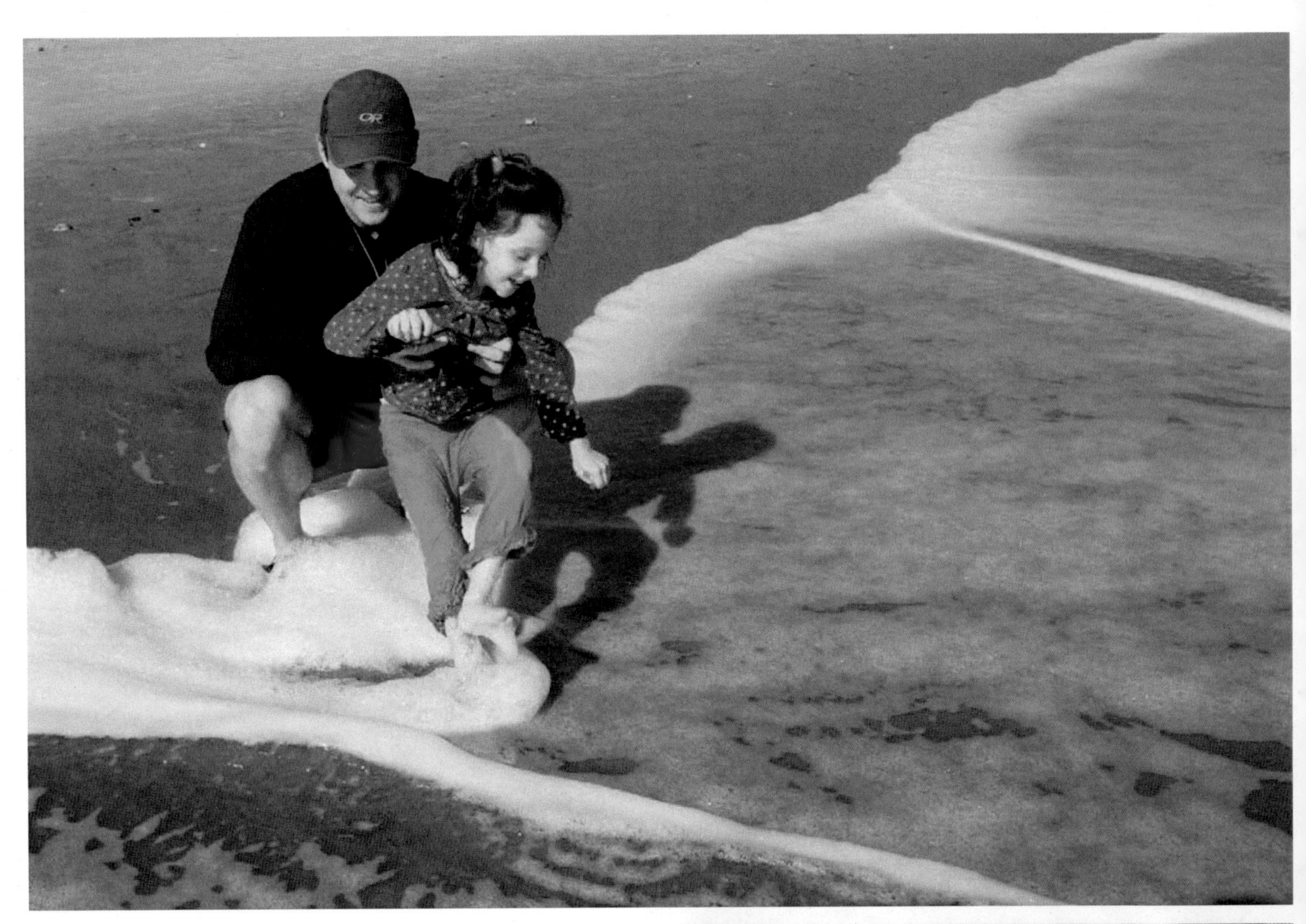

Is There a Cure for CP?

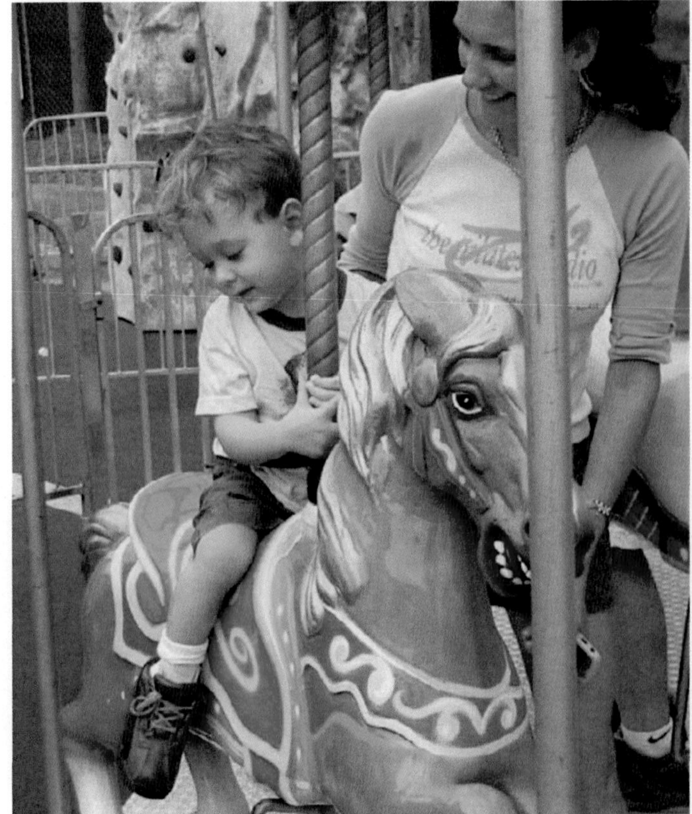

It is important to know what someone means when they ask this question. People understand CP and what it means in different ways. The CP Tool Kit presents CP as the result of an early brain injury or disturbance in early brain development with a primary focus on the problems related to movement that result. From this perspective you can't "cure" the original injury or lesion that led to CP. And at this time there is no cure for the movement disorders of CP that came from those initial events. **However, there are many different therapies, surgical interventions, medications and equipment and technology that can help reduce the symptoms of CP, its impact on the body, and improve the individual's quality of life.**

SECTION 2

Data and Statistics

THE PREVALENCE OF CP IN THE US is approximately 1 in 323 people.[2] Information about how many people have CP has been gathered by the Centers for Disease Control and Prevention (CDC) from four communities in the United States.

Currently, there is no money specifically set aside by Congress to track the numbers of people with CP. You can help researchers make progress in understanding more about the CP community by signing up for a CP registry called Cerebral Palsy Research Registry (CPRR) established by Northwestern University, the University of Chicago, and the Rehabilitation Institute of Chicago.

Here is the most recent CDC report on data collected about the CP community.

Here are the key findings from this report which is based on children who were 8 years old and living in these four communities in 2008:

- CP was more common among boys than girls.
- CP was more common among black children than white children. Hispanic and white children were about equally likely to have CP.
- Most (77%) of the children identified with CP had spastic CP.
- Over half (58%) of the children identified with CP could walk independently.
- Many of the children with CP also had at least one co-occurring condition–41% had co-occurring epilepsy.

PLEASE NOTE that the race/ethnic terminology used here is what is used on the CDC website and is used by the United States Census Bureau.

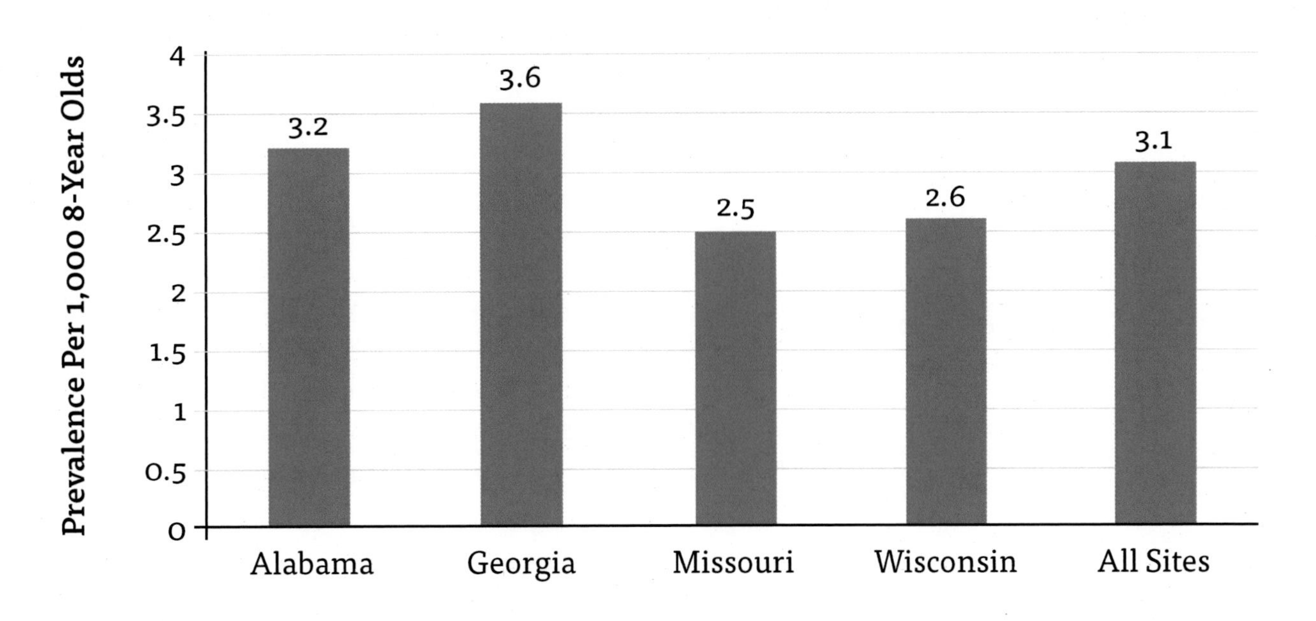

Created by the CDC National Center on Birth Defects and Developmental Disabilities 2014.

SECTION 3

Diagnosing CP

How is CP diagnosed?

RECEIVING A DIAGNOSIS OF CP is not always a straightforward path and there is no single test to determine with complete certainty that a child has cerebral palsy. Screening for CP is often done when a child has risk factors for developing cerebral palsy or when a child is delayed in meeting certain developmental milestones. **It is important to keep in mind that not all children who miss developmental milestones have CP. A CP diagnosis is often given when other diagnoses or reasons for a child's developmental delays are eliminated.**

Your child's pediatricians, developmental specialists, rehabilitation physicians, and neurologists will determine when to give your child a diagnosis of cerebral palsy and will collect the following information:

→ Observe and examine your child's movement patterns.
→ Review their medical history.
→ Evaluate their muscle tone, reflexes and posture.
→ Consider whether your child has common risk factors for cerebral palsy such as premature birth, maternal infection, multiple births, and others.
→ Ask if your child has missed multiple developmental milestones including for example, delays in rolling over, sitting independently, pulling to a stand and reaching out for objects.
→ Get your input on feeding, vision, hearing, language, cognitive functioning, behavior and social skills.

The information from those comprehensive evaluations will be considered alongside imaging of the child's brain including head ultrasounds and MRIs. Other tests may include genetic, metabolic or a combination of both.

Typically, a doctor will make the diagnosis of CP when a child is between the ages of one and three years. Some more subtle cases of CP may go undiagnosed for a longer period of time as clinicians may take additional time to rule out other diagnoses and observe the child's development. Another reason for extended periods of observation is that CP is diagnosed when motor delays persist and the child does not outgrow them. Some clinicians are beginning to use a screening tool called the General Movements Assessment as a way to try and diagnose cerebral palsy much earlier. **Regardless of when and if the diagnosis of cerebral palsy is made, it is critical that children who are considered "at risk for cerebral palsy" are identified as early as possible so they have access to support and services while the brain is still in early development.**

Receiving a diagnosis of cerebral palsy is overwhelming. However, over time and with professional guidance and support, coping with the diagnosis will become less daunting. Having a diagnosis allows you to better help your child, giving you a way to strategically organize your thoughts and actions around your child's specific problems.

Types of CP

The term cerebral palsy captures several types of movement disorders. The symptoms affect people differently including the parts of the body that are affected and to what degree. As a result, saying that someone has cerebral palsy offers little information about what challenges they do or do not face in their daily life. It also does not offer clarity about the types of treatments that may or may not be helpful.

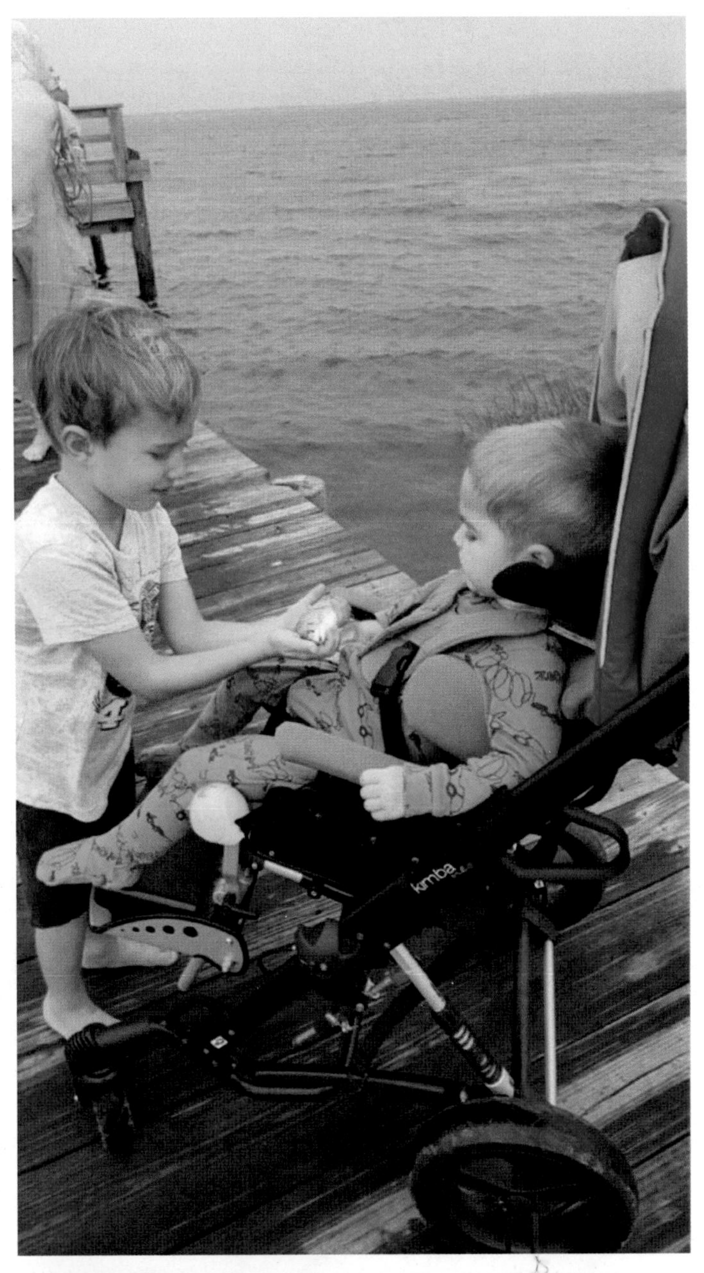

This is important information to consider when working with doctors and others who are less familiar with CP. How an individual's motor function and daily life is affected by cerebral palsy requires discussion and evaluation. **It is important to keep in mind that the initial disturbance in the brain's early development may also have affected other parts of the brain that control other functions beyond motor control** (discussed later in the Tool Kit).

Below are the most common types of CP based on the European Classifications of CP which is the most widely accepted standard for discussing cerebral palsy. **These types of cerebral palsy highlight the *primary* movement disorder that is interfering with the individual's motor control and function.** The type of CP may refer to abnormal muscle tone, involuntary movements, or both. There may also be other symptoms or other types of abnormal muscle tone that are observed and interfere with the individual's daily activities. For example, people with spastic forms of CP may also have some areas of the body that are hypotonic or "floppy."

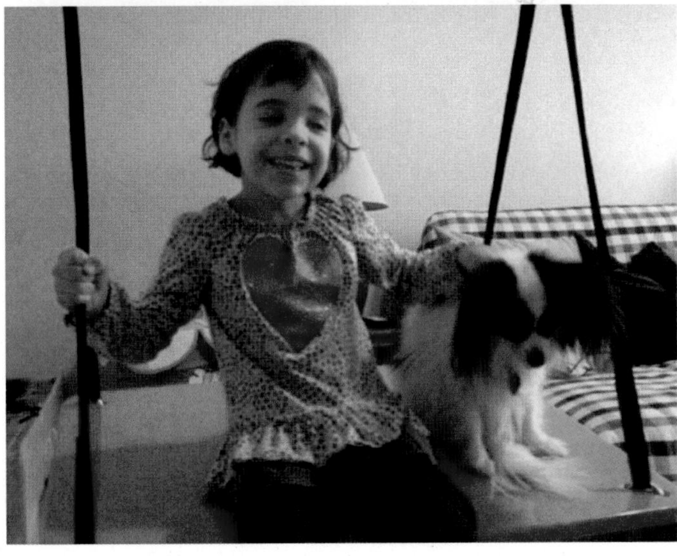

Spastic

The majority of individuals with CP have the spastic form. In spastic CP the individual has abnormal muscle tone and the muscles are stiff, making

Classifications of Spastic Type Cerebral Palsy

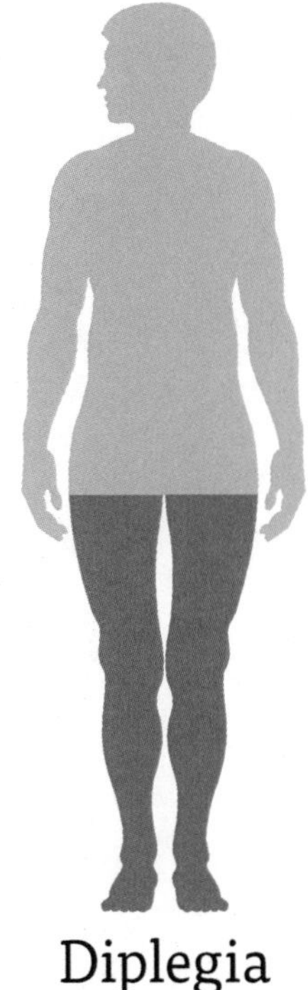

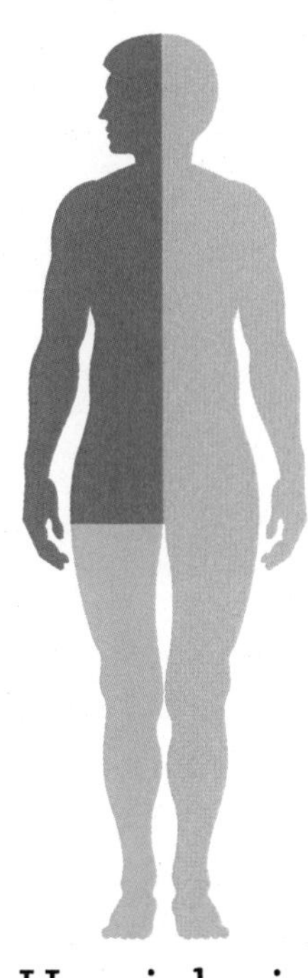

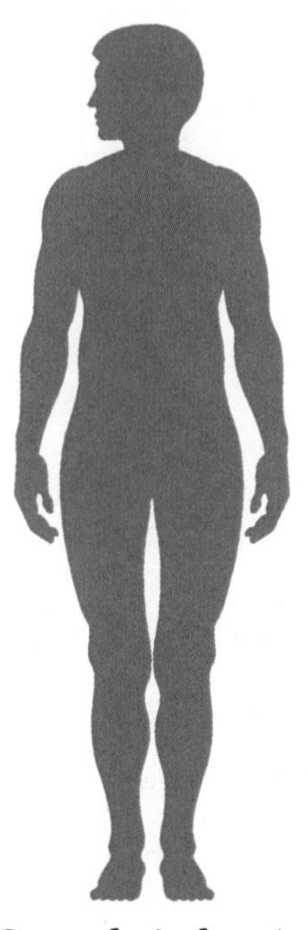

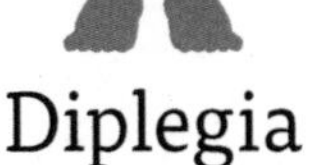

Hemiplegia

Quadriplegia

MORE LESS

movement difficult. Spastic cerebral palsy can affect specific parts of the body leaving the remaining parts unaffected or much less affected (whereas other types of CP typically affect the entire body). You may hear clinicians use the following terms that identify which parts of the body have spasticity.

HEMIPLEGIA
Mostly one side of the body is affected.

DIPLEGIA
Mostly the lower half of the body is affected.

QUADRIPLEGIA
All four limbs are affected. The muscles of the trunk, face and mouth can also be affected.

These terms are often confusing because how CP affects different parts of the body can change daily and doctors may interpret presentations differently.

Recently more researchers and clinicians have begun using the terms **bilateral** (affecting both sides-bi = two) and **unilateral** (affecting one side-uni = one) to replace the above terms in order to more generally, and perhaps more accurately describe an individual's presentation. What terms you hear depends on the preference of the physician and therapy professionals you meet.

Why the difference in opinion?
One clinician may use diplegia to describe an individual who has *less* impairment on the upper half compared with the lower half of the body, even though all four limbs are affected. This can cause confusion about how to direct treatment because a diagnosis of diplegic CP may convey that the upper part of the body does not require support or treatment. Another clinician may look at the same child, recognize this problem, and provide a diagnosis of quadriplegia.

Dyskinetic

About 10 to 20 percent have this form of CP. Dyskinetic CP is an umbrella term characterized by three different types of **involuntary movements** including **dystonic**, **athetoid**, and **choreic** (but the individual does not have to have all of them). These disorders of movement often involve the entire body and are particularly noticeable when the person begins to move, but may also occur at rest.[3] Individuals who have dyskinetic movements often have spasticity too. In these cases where two or more types of CP (i.e spastic and dyskinetic) are seen together, the individual is considered to have a mixed form of CP.

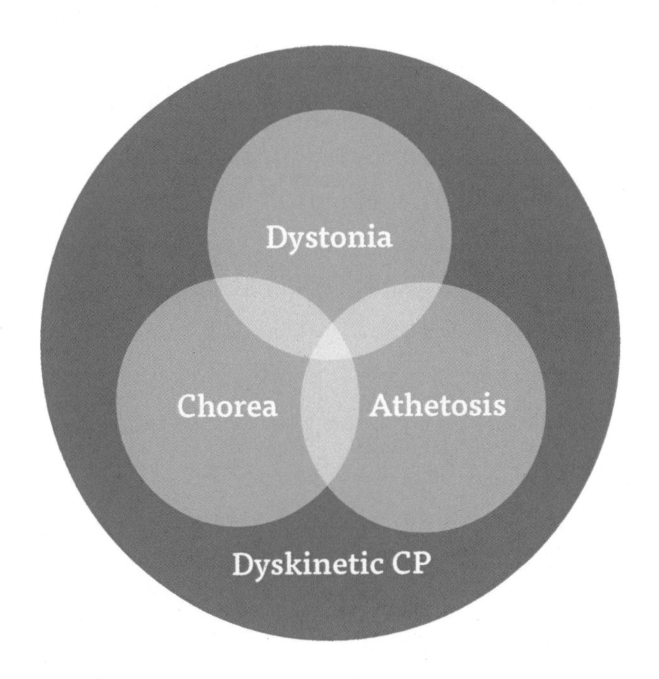

The Three Movement Disorder Types of Dyskinetic CP:

DYSTONIA—Dystonia is characterized by intermittent or lengthy muscle contractions that lead to twisting and repetitive movement sequences, abnormal posture or both. Dystonic postures are often triggered by attempts at voluntary movement.[4] Dystonia can be present in one part of the body, known as **focal dystonia**, seen during specific tasks or postures, known as **task-specific dystonia**, or throughout the whole body, known as **generalized dystonia**.

ATHETOSIS—People who have athetoid movements experience slow, continuous, involuntary twisting movements that prevent stable posture. The parts of the body that make up these movements are the same each time (unlike choreiform movements where the parts of the body involved may change).[5] The term "athetosis" comes from the Greek word meaning "without position or place" which refers to the person's inability to keep a stable posture.[6]

CHOREA—Characterised by a sequence of one or more involuntary movements that are abrupt and appear irregular. Unlike dystonic movements choreiform movements look more rapid, unpredictable, and ongoing. People with mild chorea may appear fidgety or clumsy, while those with more severe chorea have larger, more noticeable movements. Choreic movements may appear to flow randomly from one muscle group to another and may involve the trunk, neck, face, tongue, legs and arms. They may also occur with athetosis, referred to as choreoathetosis, or they may also occur with dystonic movements (see diagram to the left).[7] Choreic movements subside during sleep.

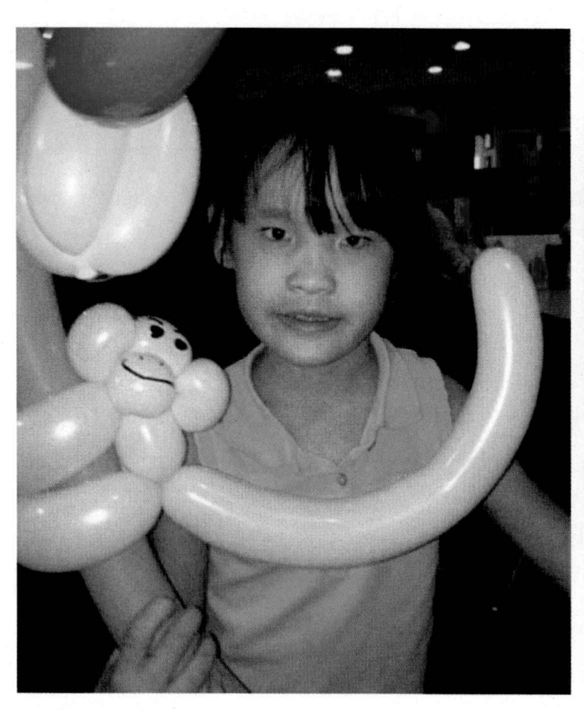

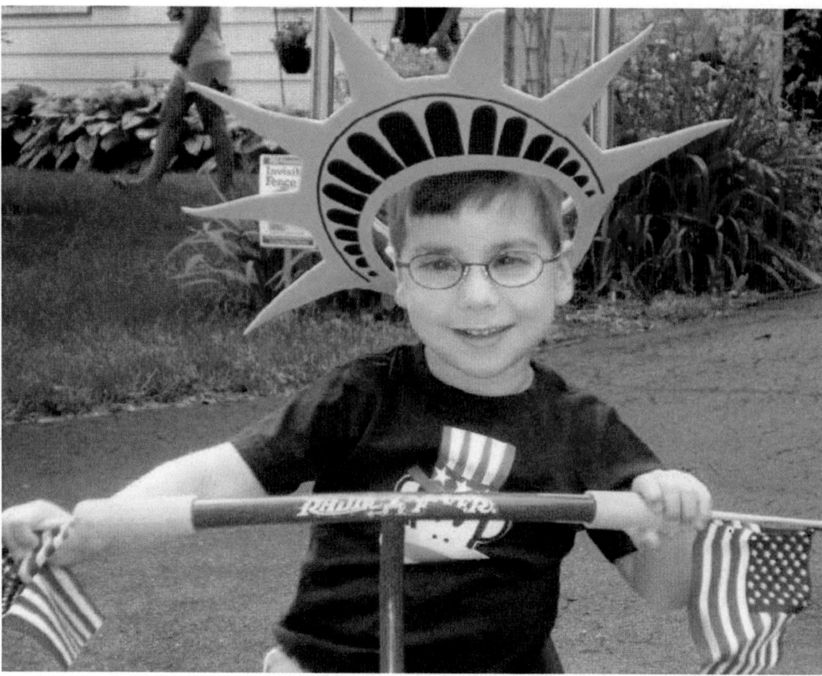

Ataxic

About 1 to 10 percent of people with CP have the ataxic form. Ataxic CP is caused by damage to the balance centers of the brain and individuals may have problems with balance, depth perception and coordination. It is often characterized by wobbly or shaky purposeful movements (occurring with the intention to move), difficulty with muscles overshooting or undershooting to meet a specific target, and may also involve difficulty coordinating precise finger movements for fine motor skills such as writing or using utensils. The word "ataxia", comes from the Greek word, " a taxis" meaning "without order or lacking coordination." Ataxia may affect any part of the body and may lead to problems with speech, swallowing and coordinating eye movements.

Mixed

These individuals present with symptoms of more than one of the previous three forms of CP. The most common mixed form includes spasticity and dyskinetic movements but other combinations are also possible.

After learning what type of CP your child has, understanding more about individual functional abilities and support needs often provides the most meaningful information for how to direct therapy and other medical interventions. The Gross Motor Function and Classification Scale, or GMFCS, is a tool often administered by a developmental pediatrician or a physical therapist. It is designed to describe an individual's present ability to move and their need for supportive devices. In addition to this and other professional assessments, it is also very important for you to share **your insight** about what you or other caregivers notice about your child's movement. The people who spend the most time with your child may notice important subtleties about how your child moves which can help your team of physicians and therapy professionals determine the most effective treatment plans.

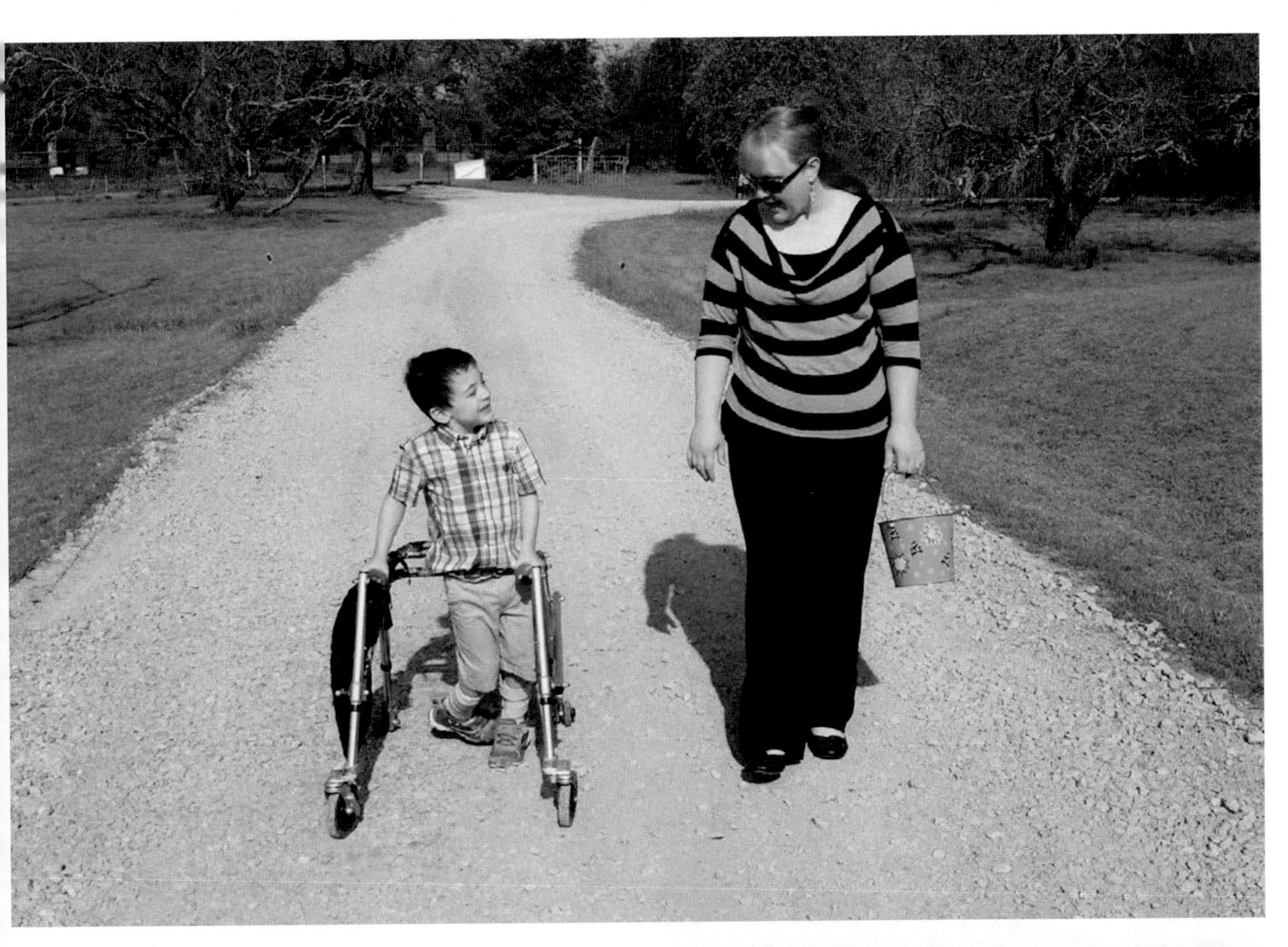

How does a CP diagnosis help your child?

A diagnosis of CP impacts many aspects of care. For example, the type of CP your child has guides treatment decisions and determines which therapies and treatments are available and recommended. In addition, a CP diagnosis signals the need for screening and monitoring for conditions that may accompany CP, such as seizures and visual impairment. Having a diagnosis also accelerates the process of getting insurance approval for medication, equipment, therapy services and/or in-home nursing care, and points you in the direction of how to help your child.

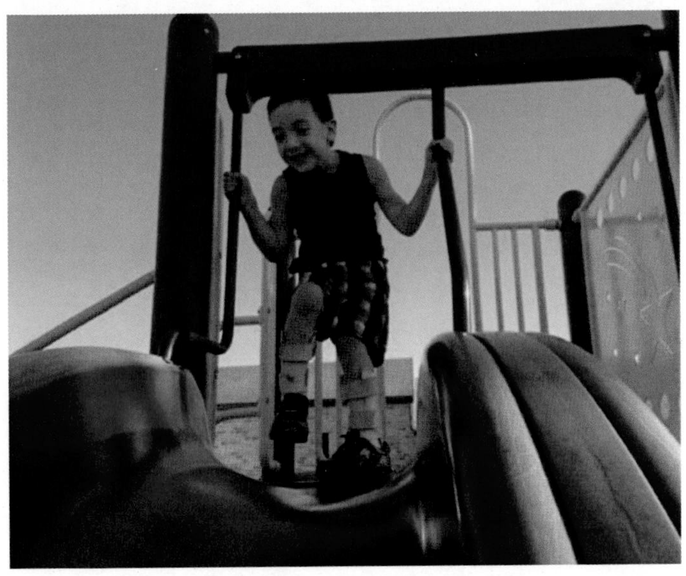

Remember a CP diagnosis does not define your child or their future. Rather, it enables you and their medical team to hone in on the specific interventions that will make a difference for your child.

Accepting a diagnosis of Cerebral Palsy

Watching your child develop and not knowing what specific problems you all may be facing together often feels scary. It is important to keep an open and positive mind about your child's development while also reaching out for the support and treatment your child may need. There is no denying that beginning this journey is hard, but with commitment to your child and determination, you will move forward. You will also discover that you have inner resources you never knew existed.

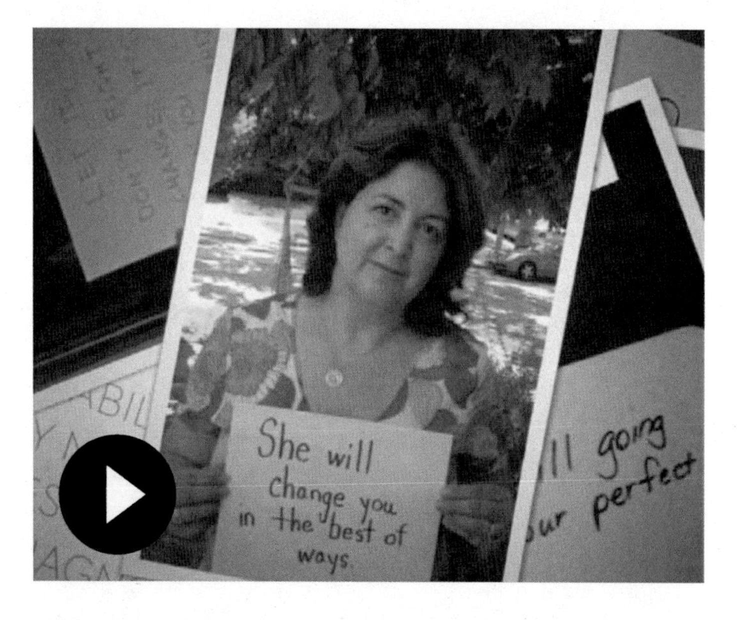

The "Extreme Parenting Video Project" organized by writer and blogger Elizabeth Aquino, is a beautiful video of what parents of children with disabilities would tell themselves if they could go back to the day their child was diagnosed.

"If I could go back to when I got the diagnosis and give myself any advice, it would be to start an exercise routine for myself. Personally, I love walking, but any movement that makes you stronger and gives you space and time to process feelings/ideas/information is important. You might have to help your children do things and/or lift heavy equipment on your own. Also, carving out even 30 minutes a day for yourself is going to be really important in the long run. I can't emphasize enough the importance of your own self-care."

Claire, Parent of Jakob, age 4

A Mom's Perspective

by Michele Shusterman

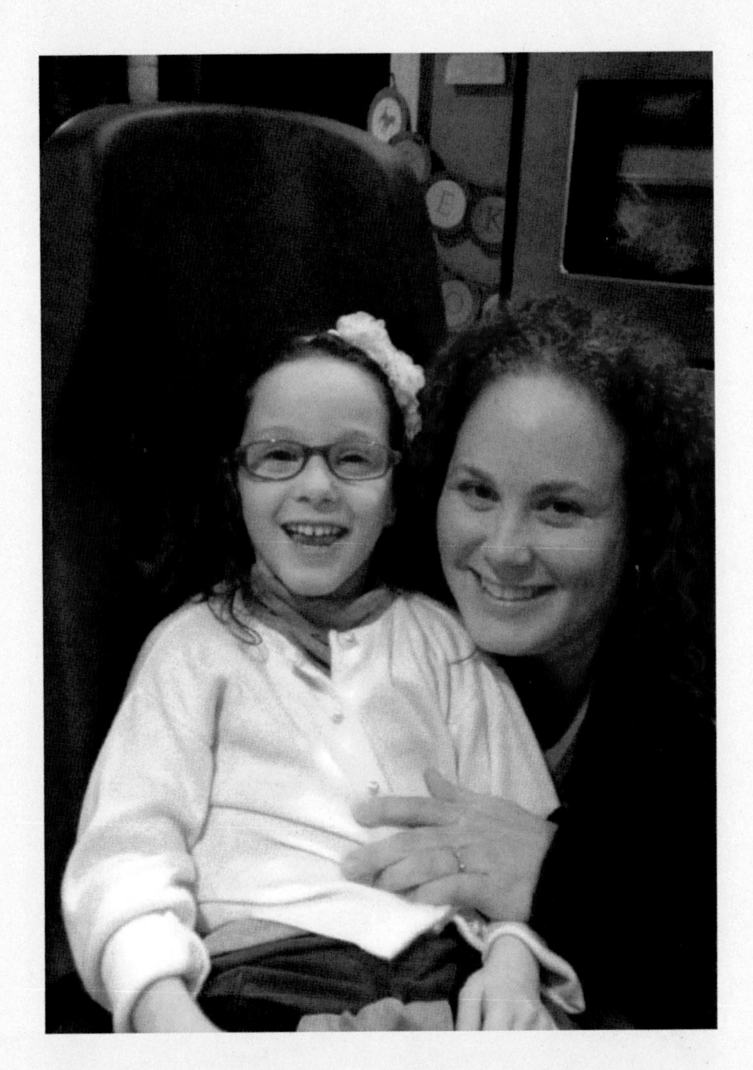

THE DAY MY DAUGHTER WAS DIAGNOSED WITH CP the doctor told me that nothing had changed. What he meant to convey was that my daughter was still the same child but now she had a name for her symptoms. But for me something did change. Receiving the diagnosis of CP was a game changer and I was frightened because it meant that my daughter would not outgrow her motor delays. Even though I had been told CP was not a progressive condition, once it had a name I felt my child had more problems than the day prior, when she didn't have the diagnosis. I was familiar with the term cerebral palsy and I recalled a childhood acquaintance who had a complex form of CP. All of the images and ideas I ever had about CP (and many were incorrect) flooded my mind and I superimposed them onto my daughter.

I needed time to process what I was feeling and thinking, including the guilt that I felt as the person who brought my daughter into the world. I needed to grieve. I needed to get comfortable with not knowing what exactly my child would be facing and what she would need from me, her mother. This "not knowing" was very hard for me to accept. I am someone who likes to know what is expected of me so that I can prepare and "conquer." As I learned more, I realized that I would not be able to prepare myself for a neatly outlined present and future, and I humbly acknowledged that I could not "conquer" cerebral palsy. However, I did learn that I could empower myself with the knowledge required to support my child and help her reach her greatest possible potential.

It is important to give yourself and each member of your family the time to process what it means to them personally. You and your spouse may have very different reactions. It may be hard to hear what one another may be feeling. Because these feelings may emerge at different times for each of you, it may be very helpful to seek counseling.

Often parents ignore their feelings of fear, shame, or guilt hoping they will quickly pass. In my experience I have learned that you cannot begin to accept your child's diagnosis by burying your feelings. True acceptance will only come when you face what you feel and think about having a loved one with CP. **Grieving is a necessary and healthy part of coping with this journey.** Once you do this it is often much easier to work toward seeing your circumstances in a new way and understanding your feelings about them.

A Dad's Perspective

by James Spinner

I REMEMBER SITTING IN THE DOCTOR'S OFFICE a few days after my daughter was born and being told that she had brain damage. My body went numb and the only thing I could think to say was "I feel like we've just been given a life-long sentence." If I could go back and give advice to that scared person in the doctor's office, I would tell him the following:

→ Over time you will go through a range of emotions, including fear, anger and sadness. It's important to allow yourself to experience all of them. I remember those early days being so hectic. The only way I knew how to get through it was to keep my head down and work as hard as possible. I woke up a few months later and realized I was still as numb as I was on that first day. I had never allowed myself to process everything that was going on, and as a result I felt isolated and bitter. Allow yourself time to go through all of these emotions and don't be ashamed of them. They are normal and healthy and are necessary for you to work through in order to be the parent that your child needs.

→ A diagnosis is not a prognosis. Every person with CP is different and no one knows what your child will be capable of doing. Don't listen to the naysayers, in fact, remove them from your life. A doctor or therapist that doesn't believe in your child's potential isn't someone you need around anyway.

→ You will be all right. Your child will love you and you will love them. You will rejoice in their accomplishments and swell with pride as they overcome their challenges. You will melt when they smile, and your heart will leap when they tell you they love you. Life will go on, and you will find moments of great joy together.

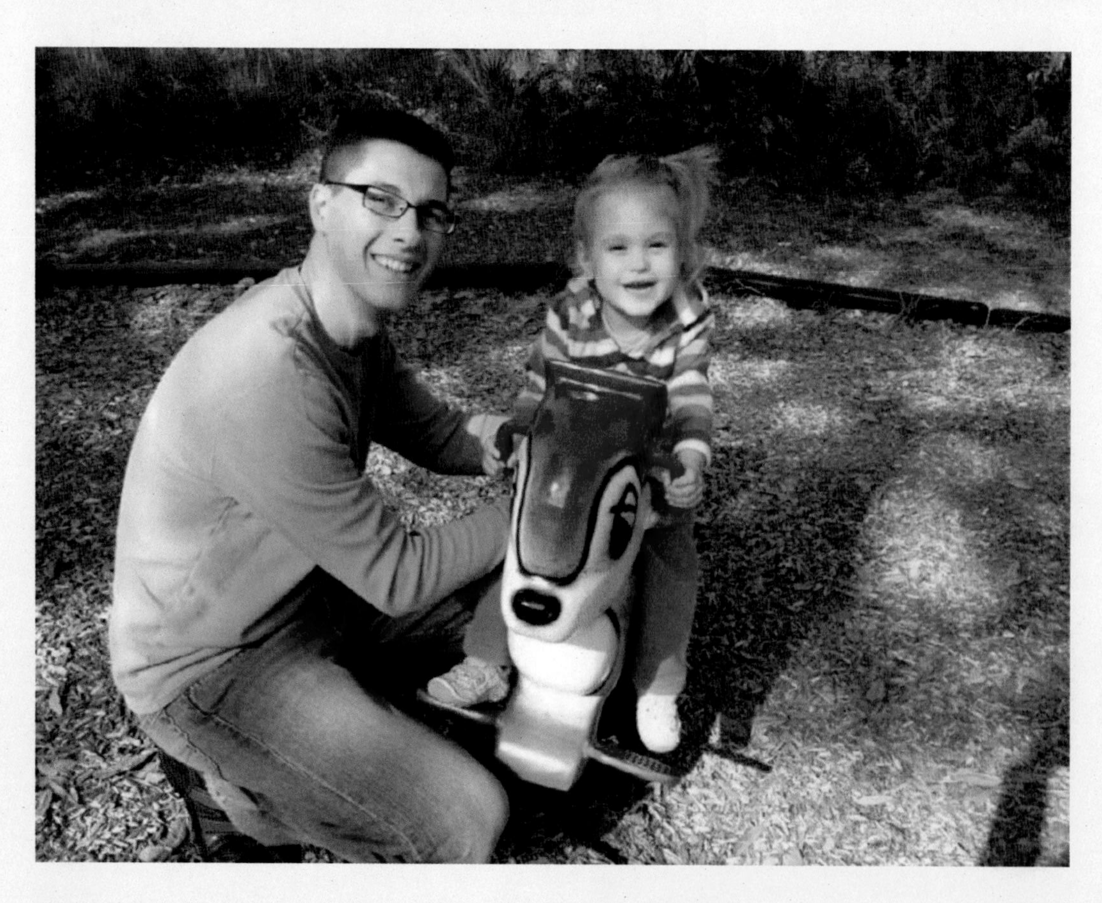

SECTION 4

Who Else Has CP?

IT IS ESTIMATED THAT SEVENTEEN MILLION PEOPLE WORLDWIDE have CP. They are librarians, activists, doctors, service providers, lawyers, actors, comedians, teachers, artists, athletes and more. Knowing that someone has a diagnosis of CP does not tell you much about their abilities, challenges, or who they are as people. Here are some individuals with cerebral palsy and their stories:

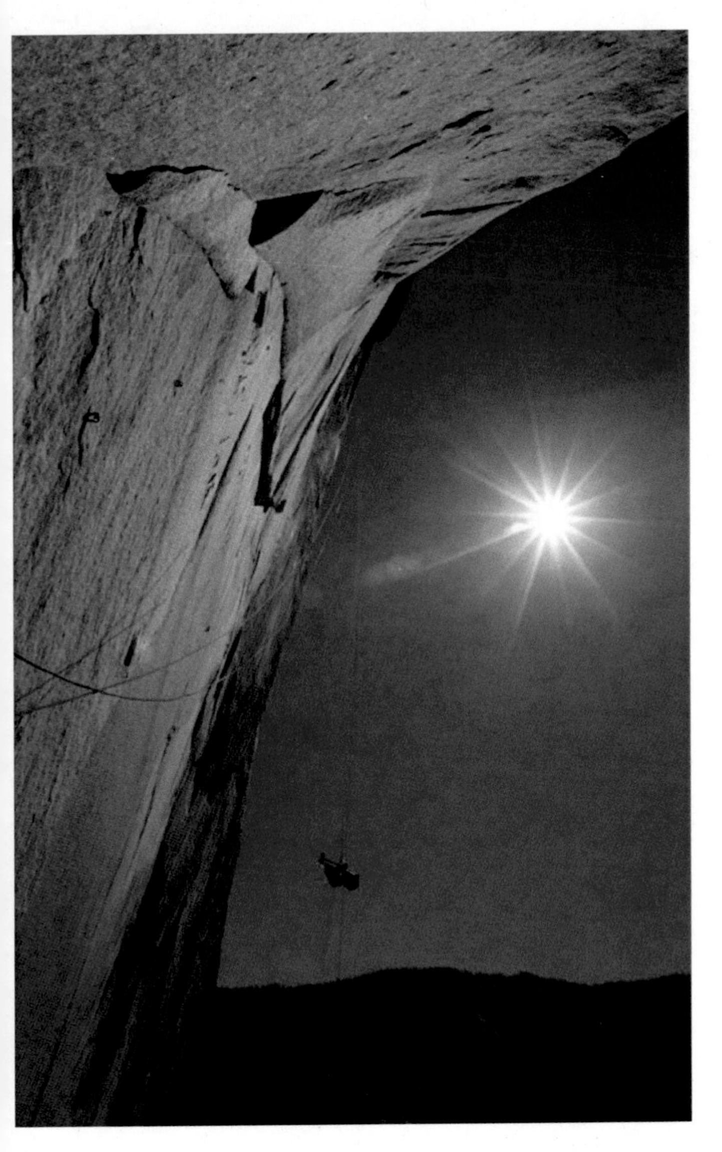

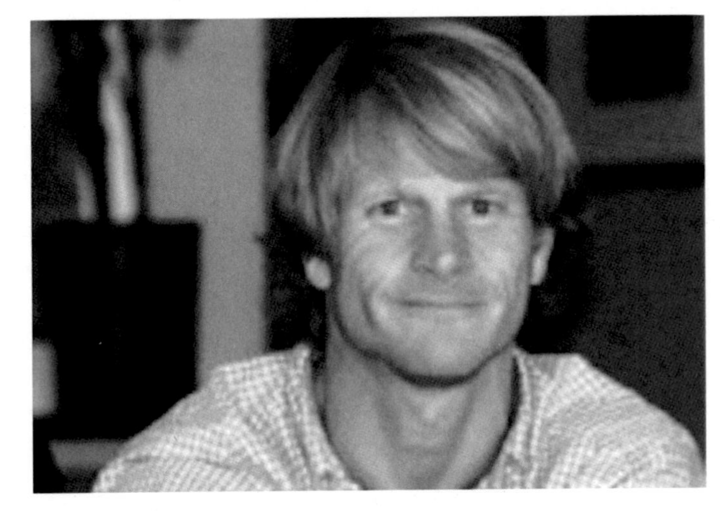

"Just because your child has CP, doesn't mean that they can't have a productive and fulfilling life."

Steve Wampler

Steve Wampler was born with a severe form of cerebral palsy. His parents worked tirelessly to integrate him into public schools as well as determine both the limits and possibilities of his future. Joe and Gayle Wampler worked with doctors and therapists, read medical journals and looked in every nook they could find in an effort to help Steve and to advance his abilities.

The year they learned about a wilderness camp in the high Sierras of California, they put him on a bus that summer. They never imagined that that camp, among all the other opportunities, would be the profound and permanent life changer that it became for him.

Here's how Steve tells it:

"Camp, summer after summer changed my whole future. It changed everything about my life, my expectations, it showed me who I could become and how. I was never again to be a person that would not be challenged, and that would not

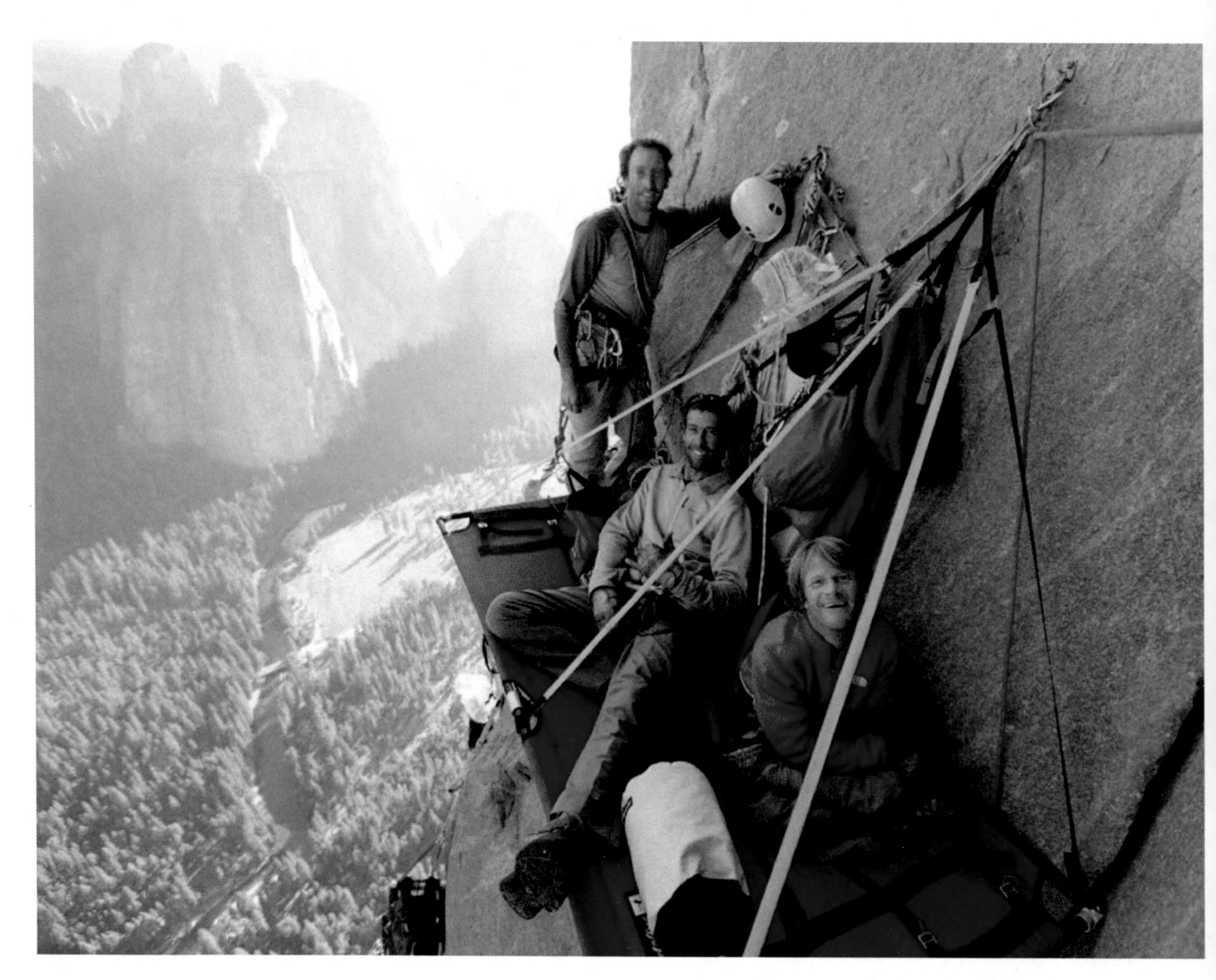

challenge myself in every aspect of my life whether it be physically, socially or in relation to who I thought I was in the world or my sense of obligation and responsibility as a man. I learned there, as a kid, that in spite of my disability, I had a place in the world, and that I was expected to contribute to my own life. Camp did all of that for me."

Steve went on to graduate from college (UC Davis) with a Bachelor of Science in Environmental Engineering (EE). He married and had two children. His life and career path were in order, yet he couldn't shake off the ever-present occupation to somehow involve himself with a camp for kids of this generation. He was so convinced that the wilderness experience would help others as it had him, that he risked it all, and went to work raising money to reopen the camp he once attended. Now reopened, Camp Wamp has been providing life-changing opportunities for hundreds of kids between the ages of 10-18 with physical disabilities since 2002.

Steve Wampler was the first person with a disability to climb El Capitan in Yosemite National Park. He wishes to inspire kids to achieve what they want in life and his climb was in their honor. It took 20,000 pull-ups, 5 nights, and 6 days on the sheer face of a mountain with the use of only one limb.

Below are some photos from that experience and a link to the film documenting Steve's amazing feat: http://www.wamplerfoundation.org/wamplersascent.html

Julius van der Wat

My name is Julius van der Wat. I am an artist and I live in Johannesburg, South Africa. When I was young, a doctor told my parents that I would never be able to speak and that they should place me in a nursing center. They ignored the doctor's' advice--something I am very happy about. I am a wheelchair user and I have a full-time shadow.

I believe I am in the chair for a purpose. I want to change people's perception of what "normal" is. I want to show that I can be as "normal" as anyone else. People with physical disabilities will be better accepted into everyday society if we are seen more often. During the week I work as a computer assistant at Helpmekaar College in Johannesburg. Work gives me a goal in life and it is a place where I mean something.

The Apple iPad also drastically changed my life. I use a computer pen that is fastened to my helmet to paint with on the iPad screen. I had no creative outlet before discovering the Ipad and it is very therapeutic. I can paint, Facebook, read books and I can even do my own banking now. Life can be tough at times but how you experience it depends on your attitude. God doesn't make mistakes, I am as normal as anyone out there.

Emily W.

The first doctor I had told my mom that I needed to be institutionalized, and that I would never be more than a dog that she could train to do tricks!! Well, my parents didn't listen, but did teach me a LOT of tricks!! I completed high school (on time!!). I was mainstreamed with two hours of special education. I went to college and received a degree in elementary education. I also attended graduate school, and received a master's degree in curriculum and instruction. I obtained additional certifications in library science, instructional technology, and supervision. I started working (something doctors didn't think was possible), and wasn't satisfied with one master's, so I completed an online master's degree in library science. I am in my eighth year at a middle school where I began as a librarian and I am now the computer lab manager. I LOVE my job because achievements mean more when you have to struggle for them. I think I've proven to the personnel director that I CAN run a library and a computer lab!!

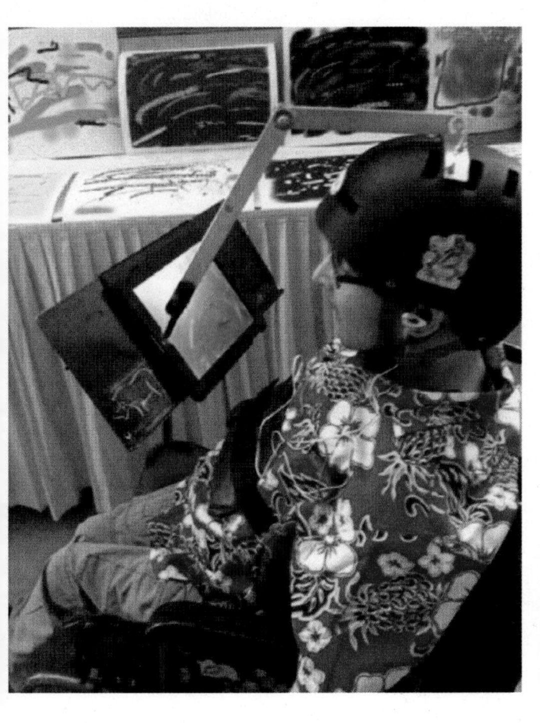

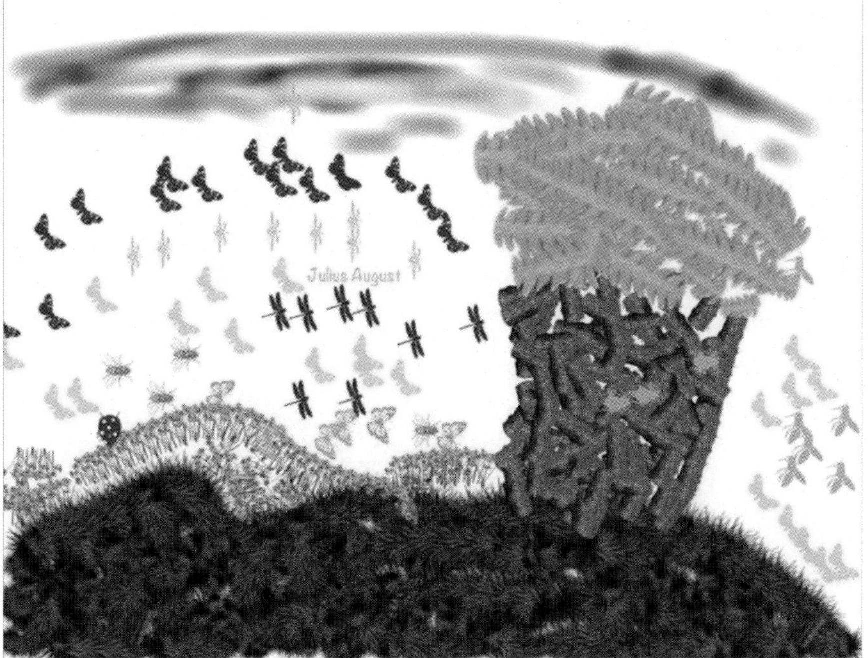

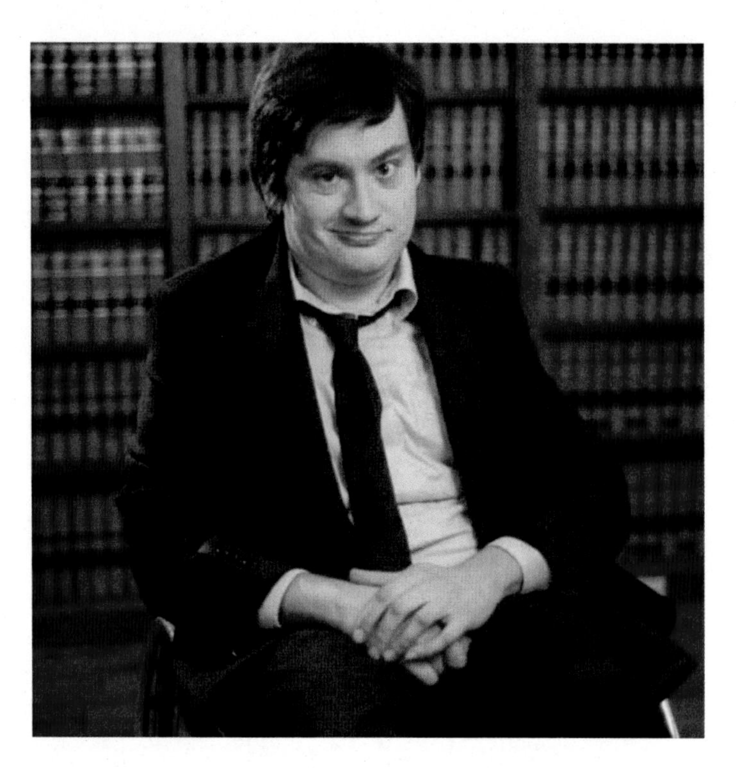

Ralph Strzalkowski, Esq, JD, LL.M

When I was born, I was so tiny and fragile, the doctors told my parents to prepare for the worst. The first twenty-four hours were supposed to be telling—then forty-eight, then seventy-two. My parents put together my baptism in a hurry, an unusual feat in then communist Poland. Thirty-five years later, I'm still here. And I wish I could tell my mom and dad from back then that their years of hard work and dedication paid off. They'd be thrilled to see my life today and I know it would have given them some comfort.

My parents carried me to school every day to offer me the regular, most "normal" school experience, up the stairs as most Polish facilities at the time didn't have elevators and people with disabilities were not welcome at all. From a regular elementary school to a more competitive math-physics profiled high school class, I proved to be a really good student. At the same time, we tried every CP rehabilitation method my mom could get her hands on. My parents pushed me hard and never gave up on me. That drive and motivation became a part of who and how I am as well.

In 1998 I was accepted to Warsaw University Law. I managed to maintain my scholarship through most of it and graduated summa cum laude. But the outside world of the now capitalist Poland wasn't much more welcoming and I wanted to try and see if I could live differently. I came to America for one year to complete an academic program. Two programs and ten years later I'm a practicing attorney. "Never, never quit"- my life's philosophy became the title of my 2013 book published in London, supporting a local CP charity.

I now practice law in Florida and DC and run a local charity called Florida Disability Access and Awareness Foundation, that pushes for more accessibility. I live in Gainesville where I was named one of the city's eighteen most interesting people in 2010.

R. Strzalkowski, Esq, JD, LL.M
Attorney at Law

Dartania Emery

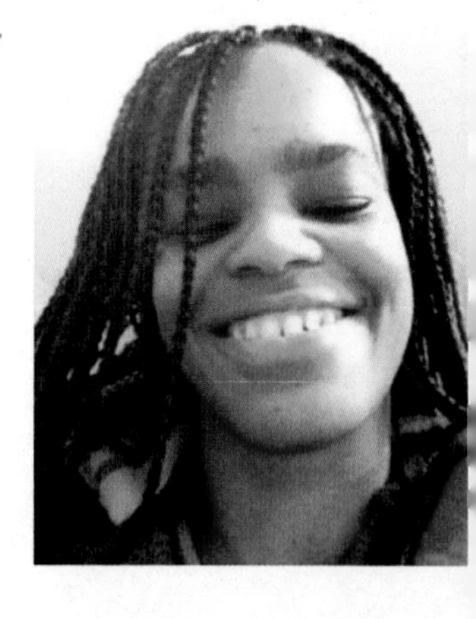

My name is Dartania Emery. I'm twenty-seven years old. I have spastic diplegic CP. I have 3 other siblings--one older brother and two younger sisters. I got my bachelor's degree in sport management in 2011. I've lived on my own since around the same year. I use an electric wheelchair, a manual wheelchair and a walker to get around. I've volunteered as a museum tour guide with the local history museum since 2014. I love music, books and watching crime shows on television. I've never let the CP define me or get in the way of things I want to do in life.

Kathleen Friel, PhD

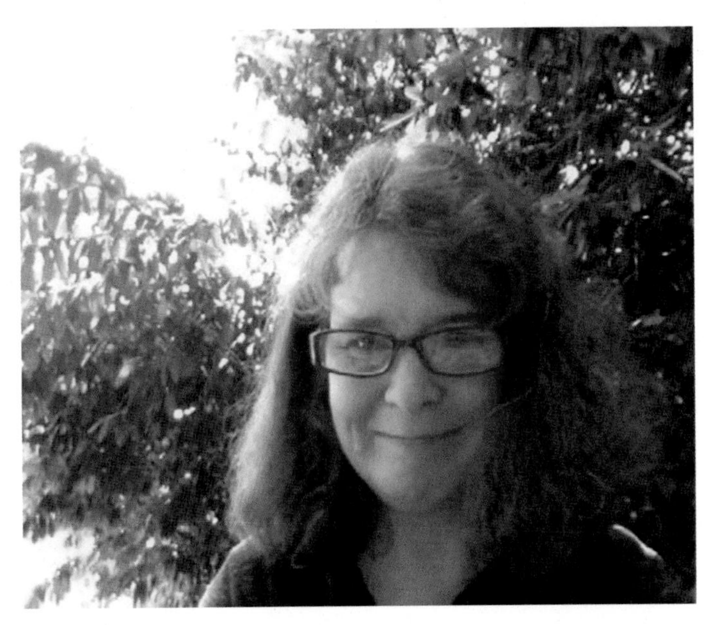

When I was first diagnosed with cerebral palsy at around two years of age, the neurologist told my parents that I had very little potential for improvement. I am so grateful that my parents ignored that prognosis and continually encouraged me to embrace life. Despite my childhood hatred of anyone who had anything to do with medical care, I became fascinated with the complex beauty of the nervous system. In college and in graduate school, I developed a passion for research. In 2002, I earned a doctorate in neurophysiology, with a focus on understanding how the brain responds to injury and rehabilitation. I then completed a research fellowship, during which I studied the development of movement, with an eye toward understanding the best ways to restore movement after a developmental brain injury.

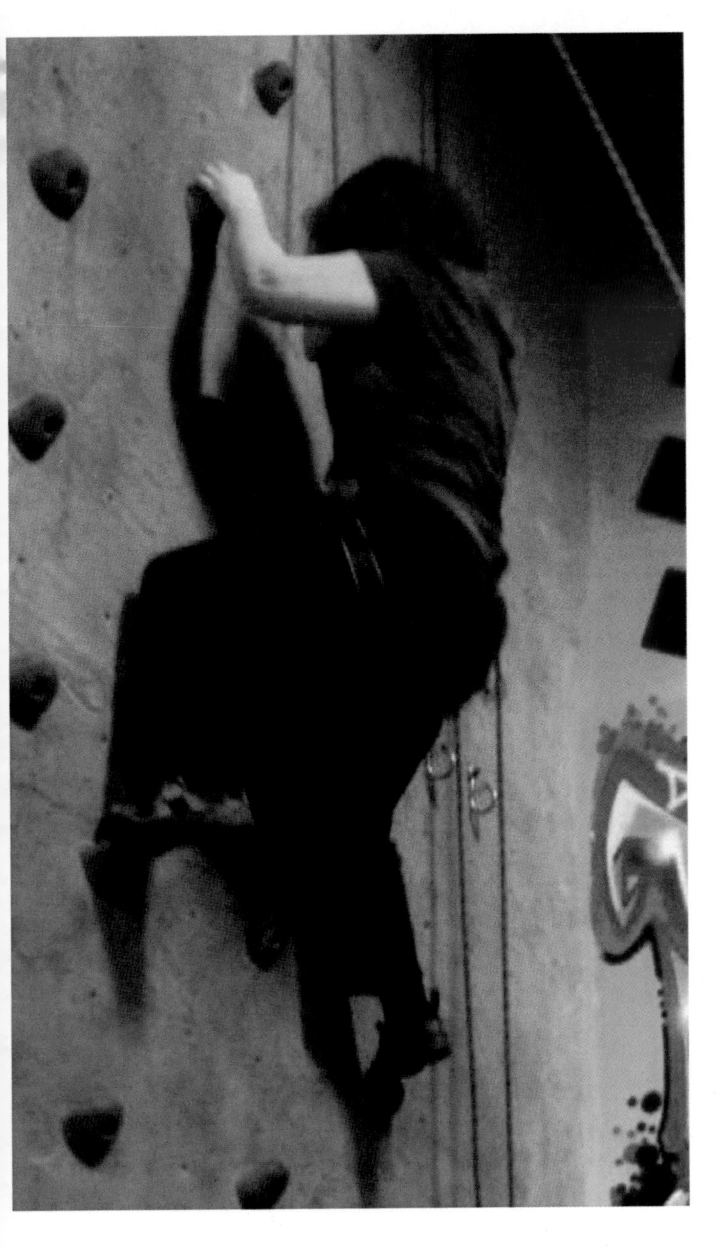

In 2013, I was hired by the Burke-Cornell Medical Research Institute to start a research program for children with cerebral palsy. In my laboratory, we use non-invasive brain stimulation to understand brain function in kids with CP. Our goal is to develop new, more effective therapies for children and adults who have CP. Our findings indicate that skillful, repetitive movements can not only improve movement in people with CP, but can also strengthen the brain networks that control movement. In 2014, I was named a "Pioneering Woman in Technology" by the Westchester County Association. My work has received federal funding since 1998 and has been honored with several scientific awards.

My abiding interest in movement follows me when I leave the lab! I have practiced taekwondo since 2011, which has greatly improved my strength, flexibility, and stamina. Despite weak limbs — and a mild fear of heights — I also enjoy adaptive rock climbing.

SECTION 5

After the Diagnosis—Creating Your Child's Team

Coordinating Care

CP IS A COMPLICATED CONDITION. No two children with CP have exactly the same strengths and needs. Your child's care needs will change over time. In addition to their primary care doctor, they will need visits with other pediatric specialists. They may need other health–related services such as nutrition care, dental care, glasses, braces and other equipment. They will see an alphabet soup of professionals from different disciplines, including PT, OT, SLP (Speech and language pathologists/therapists), EIS (Early intervention services), and IEP (Individualized Education Plan) teams. Finding your way in such a complex web of services and coordinating your child's care can be overwhelming at times. Nobody expects you to do it alone, and there are important resources to help you along the way.

The single most helpful resource for you should be your child's primary care medical home; the place from which all other care is organized. Your child's primary care provider (whether pediatrician, family physician, nurse practitioner or physician assistant) is part of a practice that is striving to be your child's medical home. They want to provide care that is **family-centered**, comprehensive, continuous, accessible, accountable and coordinated. This kind of care is extremely valuable for children with special needs and their families, and can be achieved through communication, teamwork and trust.

In family-centered care "the family is viewed as central in a child's life and the parents are seen as having the greatest insight into a child's abilities and needs."[8] The service team also considers the needs and concerns of the parents and siblings in order to ensure the family will successfully support the child's treatment program.

The cornerstones of successful family-centered care are:

- → Open information exchange
- → Respect and support for the family's wishes and preferences
- → Partnership between the family and service providers (rather than a dictatorial "take-it-or-leave-it" approach)

Not only does a family-centered approach to care result in higher satisfaction among parents, it improves outcomes for the child, parents, and entire family.[9]

IF YOU HAVE ACCESS TO A CHILDREN'S HOSPITAL that has specialized clinics for children with CP, you may be able to receive care from a team of CP specialists, e.g., orthopedic surgeon, neurologist, developmental pediatrician, physiatrist (physical medicine and rehabilitation doctor), physical therapist, orthotist, and nutritionist. Such a team may provide "one stop shopping" rather than having to visit all the specialists separately. Ideally, the team will include a social worker or care coordinator who is there to assist you in organizing your future visits and address your need for

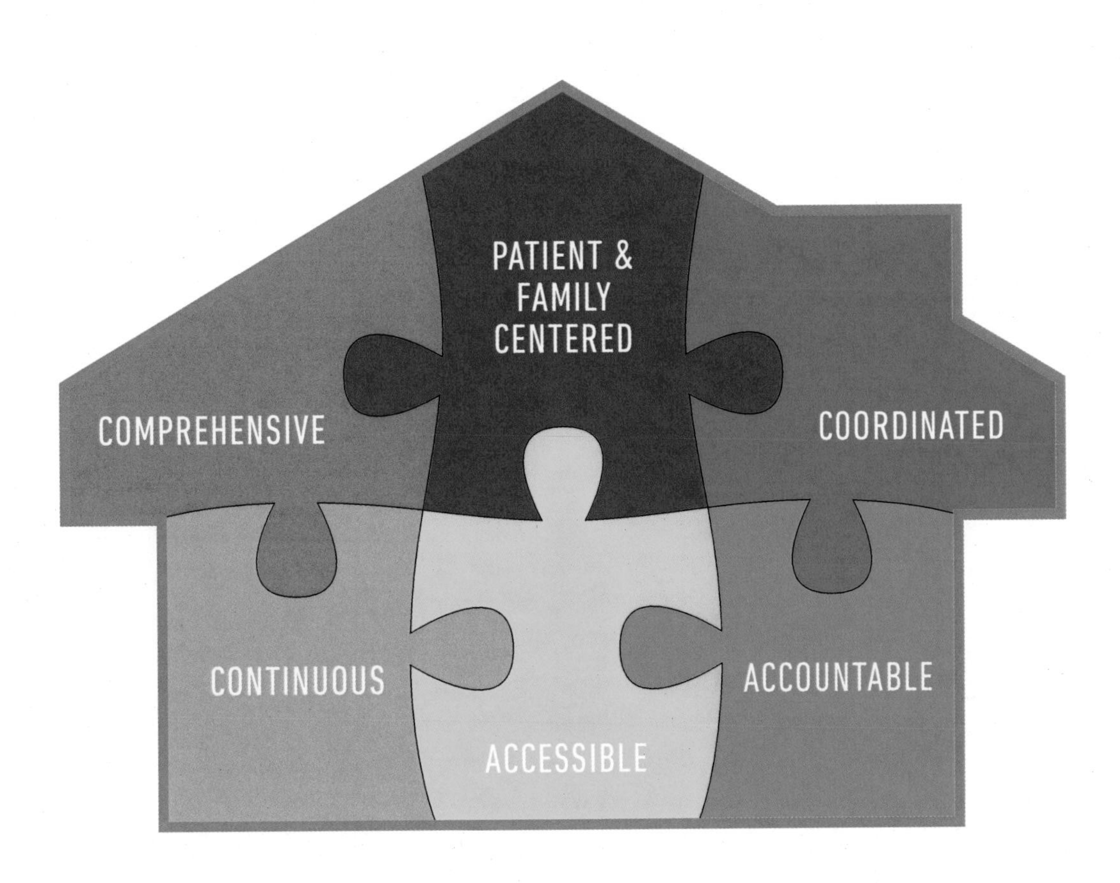

services and information. The specialty team will communicate with the child's primary care doctor about their insights and treatment plans.

IF YOU DO NOT HAVE ACCESS TO A CP CLINIC you will want to find a pediatrician who has an interest in and experience with caring for children with CP. It is helpful to interview several physicians, to best understand how care coordination will be provided through their practice. For example, you may want to ask about the different hospitals, clinics and therapists that they prefer to refer to or use, and how they will communicate together about your child's treatment plans.

The complex care needs of your child newly diagnosed with CP may feel overwhelming. Remember that putting together your child's team does not all have to be done urgently. **Care coordination is a process that unfolds over the course of many years.** Think of it in phases (that may overlap and occur more than once in your child's life at times of transition).

PHASE I: GATHERING AND UNDERSTANDING INFORMATION—about CP, about resources in your community, and about treatment options that may be right for your child.

PHASE II: BUILDING YOUR TEAM—the professionals who help to take care of your child and whom you come to trust.

PHASE III: FOCUSING ON PRIORITIES AND GOALS.

Here are some things to remember as you embark on your care coordination journey:

Take a deep breath—care needs are usually not urgent, and you have time to gather information and build your child's care team.

You are the expert on your child—You will rely on the experience of trusted experts, but you know your child best, and the experts will come to rely on you to tell them about his or her specific needs.

Your child needs a primary care medical home—Develop a trusting relationship with your child's primary care doctor, and talk constructively with the practice to help achieve the medical home.

It's all about function and participation in life—When you are evaluating treatment options and goals, think in practical terms about what will help your child to move, to communicate, to play, to learn and to do things at home, in school and in the community.

Participate in decision-making—Shared decision-making rests on asking questions and having discussions with your child's team.

Maintain a well-organized record—A file that includes test results (like brain MRI), specialist consultation reports, hospital discharge summaries, developmental evaluations, medication lists, growth chart, and contact information for your child's team members helps with care coordination.

Intensity matters, but more is not necessarily better—There are times when intensive treatment is needed to achieve goals, but if you are feeling overscheduled with different treatment visits, your child probably feels it too.

It helps when parents and different professionals speak the same language—Kids do better when professionals from different disciplines understand each other, and when medical jargon is explained in clear language. If you don't understand the terminology your team is using, ask them to explain it in different terms.

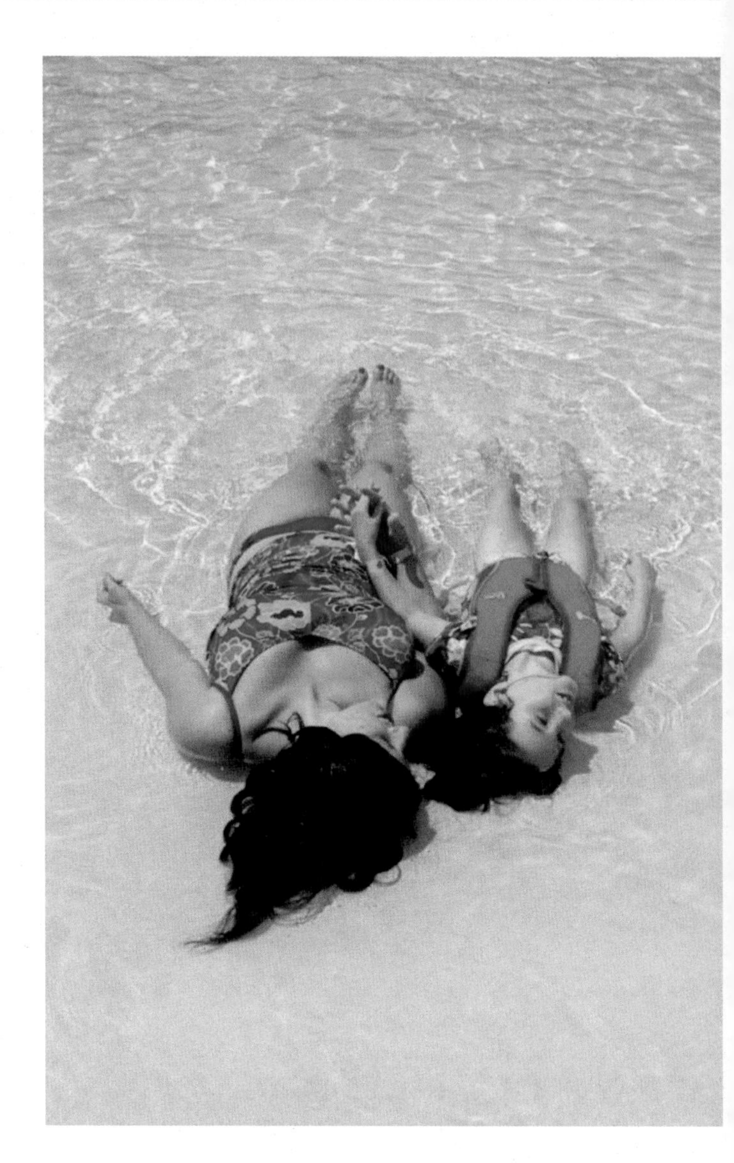

Find the right balance and take care of yourself—You are a devoted parent of a child with CP, but you may also be a husband, a wife, a student, an employee, an entrepreneur, a musician, a chef, an athlete and a host of other things. It is important to nurture and explore your interests and talents outside of parenting your child with CP.

A Parent's Perspective on Coordinating Care

Many parents may benefit from focusing their energy on becoming a well informed advocate/case manager for their child because it is an area where parents clearly have some control in making a difference in their child's development. You may have case managers as part of an early intervention program, and if you are lucky you will have the same one for a couple of years. **But you are THE ultimate case manager and advocate for your child.**

Whether you are happy with your therapists and doctors and find them competent and effective, or you disagree with how a professional approaches your child's care, your voice plays a critical role in deciding the direction of your child's care. If you are unhappy with something, you have the right to change it. If you are just beginning this journey, it may seem like a daunting responsibility. Give yourself time to find your voice, educate yourself, and observe your child. Your insight is often the most powerful tool you have to help your child. A good doctor or therapist will want to know what you see and perceive and will view your input as an integral tool to designing your child's treatment plan.

How to Provide Comfortable Care for My Child

Have you taken your child to see the doctor, therapist, or other professional and wished you could quickly debrief them on how to make your child feel comfortable during his/her visits? Perhaps someone new is on staff, or is filling in, and you would like them to have this information ahead of time.

You can use the following form to help your professional team understand more about how to make your child feel comfortable during visits:

→  How to Provide Comfortable Care for ______________.

→  OUR SAMPLE DOCUMENT How to Provide Comfortable Care for Maya.

Having a pediatrician you trust and respect is very important. They should be able to provide you with referrals to local agencies, specialists (neurologists, developmental physicians, rehabilitation physicians or CP clinics), and/or point you in the right direction for beginning this journey. **Your pediatrician will be your launching point for creating a team of doctors who will support your child; so do not be afraid to change pediatricians if you do not feel you have the right person working with you and your child.**

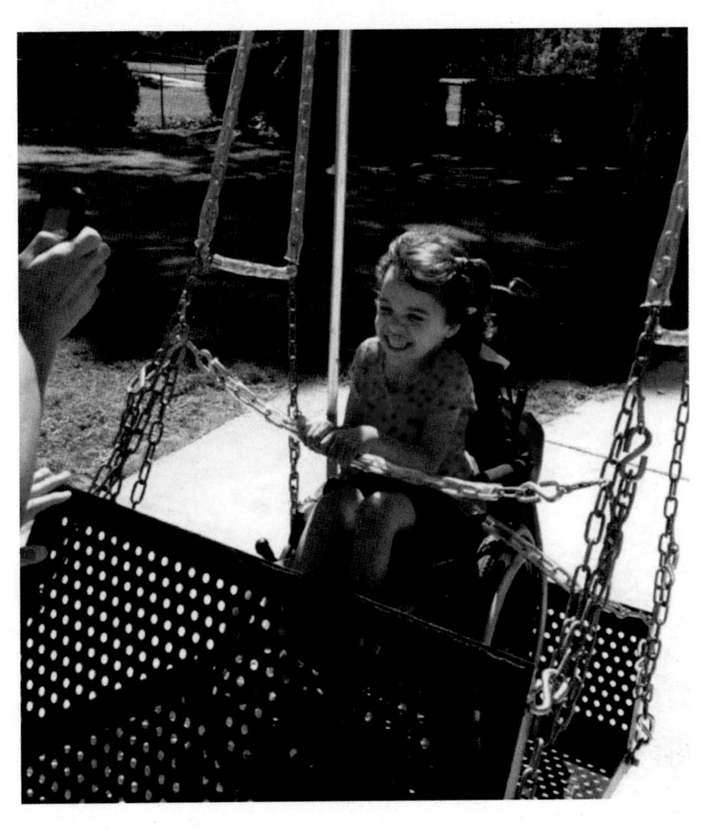

Early Assessments and Screenings

AFTER RECEIVING THE CP DIAGNOSIS your physicians and therapy professionals will continue to use developmental milestone timelines and other assessments to understand how your child is developing and where support and intervention may be needed. Evaluations, especially those that compare children to their same-age peers are often upsetting to parents because their children are developmentally behind their peers. But keep in mind that this information is being used to identify and understand how to best support your child's ongoing development, direct interventions/treatments and, in turn, maximize their participation in daily activities.

The following are a variety of assessments/screenings that may be used to evaluate and better understand different aspects of your child's development and wellbeing. What is included here is not necessarily an exhaustive list for your child. If you have concerns about an aspect of your child's health and development be sure to bring those concerns to the attention of your pediatrician and professional team.

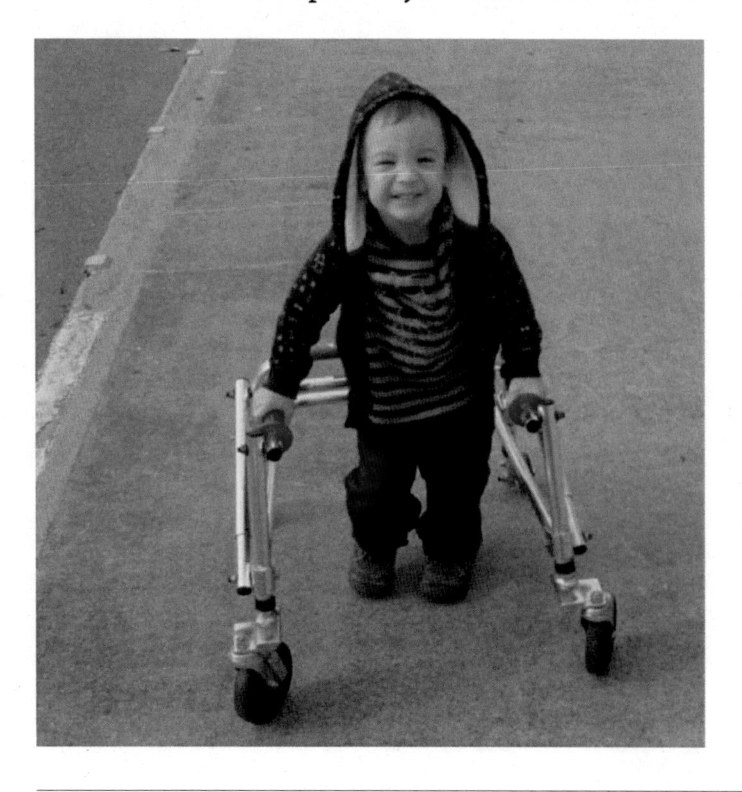

Children with CP have their own developmental timelines and your child's present conditions do not dictate their future. As a parent, it is important to focus on the progress your child is making, not the specific measurements of these tests. Celebrate your child's achievements no matter how big or small. Every milestone is a building block to another.

Movement

CONTRACTURES — A term used to describe when muscles, ligaments, and tendons become fixed in a rigid and shortened position. As motor development is delayed or does not progress in CP, muscle growth fails to keep up with the growth of the bones, so that tight muscles gradually become too short relative to the length of the bones. The increased tension in these tissues limits the individual's range of motion and may cause deformities in the bones. Contractures are usually screened for on a routine basis (typically at least every 6–12 months) by your physician and/or therapist by observing the child's movements and measuring the range of motion of their joints.

FINE MOTOR — Refers to the use of small muscle groups within the hand or wrist. Examples: grasping a small tool or writing. The Manual Ability Classification System (MACS) describes how children with cerebral palsy use their hands to handle objects in daily activities. MACS describes five levels of fine motor ability for ages 4-18. In September of 2015 Mini-MACS was developed for children under 4 years of age. The MACS levels are based on the children's self-initiated ability to handle objects and their need for assistance or adaptation to perform manual activities in everyday life. A child with no fine motor problems would be scored at "level 1" whereas a child unable to use their hands would be scored at "level 5".

GROSS MOTOR — Gross motor evaluations look at the use of large muscle groups. Examples: crawling or reaching for objects. The Gross Motor Function Classification System (GMFCS) is a five level classification system that **describes** the gross motor function of children and youth with cerebral palsy. It was designed to encourage the use of a more meaningful universal common language when discussing how cerebral palsy affects a person's mobility in daily life. The intention of the GMFCS is to focus on what people can do and move away from terms such as "mild", "moderate", "severe" which are limiting and used without any objective measure.

The descriptions used in the GMFCS describe ***general patterns of movement*** and the child's *present abilities* and *typical function*, rather than their best performance. The GMFCS levels are not intended to describe all aspects of a child's functional abilities or potential for improvement, especially at a young age. **Using the GMFCS is very helpful for setting individual goals**, establishing timelines for hip surveillance, evaluating treatments and understanding research about cerebral palsy. Ask your developmental pediatrician, physiatrist or therapy professional for more information.

Genetics

Many cases of cerebral palsy are related to easily identified risk factors such as prematurity, a lack of blood flow to the developing brain, or infection during development. However, not all children with CP have these risk factors. For these children, the development of their CP may be related to genetics, even if there is no family history of the condition.

What do you mean, "genetic"?
The 20,000 genes that make up our human genome contain the instructions that tell our bodies how to develop and function properly. Differences between one person's genes and another's help determine the body's basic characteristics, ranging from simple things like hair and eye color to more complex traits such as temperament. Such differences in the genetic code from one person to another are referred to as "genetic variants."

Sometimes a change arises in the genetic code that causes disease. This type of change is referred to as a "mutation." Genetic tests evaluate your child's DNA to look for these mutations.

How do I know if my child may have a genetic form of CP?
If the cause of your child's CP is not clear, genetic testing could offer more information. A simple blood draw is used to collect the DNA needed for this analysis.

Several different kinds of genetic mutations may lead to CP, and different methods are required to detect them. Given the complex landscape of genetic testing, it is helpful to have the guidance of a physician knowledgeable about genetic causes of CP, as well as a genetic counselor who is a professional trained to interpret and discuss the implications of genetic findings.

Identifying a genetic cause of a child's CP is important for several reasons:

- → Families may gain a better sense of what their child's future will look like and doctors may be better equipped to prevent problems before they arise.
- → Understanding what caused a child's CP can provide a sense of closure for family members who might otherwise blame themselves for their child's condition.
- → Ongoing research may identify new treatment options for children with genetic forms of CP.
- → Although rare, some forms of CP may run in families.

Growth & Nutrition

Children with cerebral palsy often grow more slowly than their more typically developing peers. Sometimes this signifies a health problem that needs to be addressed and other times the slower growth is okay for a child with CP. **Most children with CP whose growth raises concerns have problems with either feeding, severe motor impairment, or both.** Children who have problems with feeding may get less nutrition than their body needs, and children who have severe motor impairments engage much less in the movement, play and exercise that supports muscle and bone growth. Growth problems in children who have CP may also be due to genetic differences or prenatal factors. The challenge is sorting out these issues for your child and determining what may need to be addressed.

Evaluation of Growth and Nutritional Status

When children go to their pediatrician, their weight, height (standing) or length (lying), and head circumference are measured and plotted on a growth chart that compares them to typically growing children of the same age. Children who do not grow as expected on this chart attract their doctor's attention. When this happens, the doctors, dieticians and others investigate whether the child has a problem (like under-nutrition) that needs attention.

For children with CP, particularly as they get older, reliable measurements of height and weight can be difficult to obtain. If they cannot stand by the age of 2 or 3, they have often outgrown the use of standard scales for younger children and instead require specialized equipment to weigh and measure them. These scales may only be available at larger children's hospitals or specialized centers. Children with CP also may have contractures or scoliosis that make it difficult or even impossible to accurately measure their length (since these conditions affect the ability to lie straight).

When accurate measures cannot be taken or additional information is needed for growth assessment, there are a couple of alternative measurements that can provide helpful insight. To estimate height, a trained professional may measure specific areas of the body that can be used to estimate overall height (i.e. knee height or measuring length from elbow to wrist). To determine if a child's weight is appropriate for their body size, dieticians also may use skinfold measurements—measurements of the fat under the skin. Since both of these approaches are less practiced than traditional measures, it is critical that a clinician who is experienced in evaluating growth and nutrition in CP interprets the information. Only an experienced professional can determine what these values mean and how this information will be used to make decisions about the child's nutritional status.

Feeding problems

Feeding, eating, drinking and swallowing are complicated. Every swallowed bite of food or drink passes just over the airway. Eating and swallowing requires significant coordination in order to prevent aspiration of food contents into the lungs. Children with CP may have multiple issues that interfere with this process. Some of these include decreased coordination of the mouth, tongue and throat (oral motor dysfunction or "dysphagia") to manage various foods and liquids, inability to hold the head up, difficulty aligning the head with the neck and trunk to sit up, and trouble reaching for food or drink with their hands. In addition, some children with CP have other medical issues that complicate learning how to eat, such as chronic lung disease, congenital heart disease, short gut, gastroesophageal reflux, and even constipation.

Parents are usually the first to notice feeding problems. The most common symptoms in children who have difficulty feeding are

Feeding Support

Even with advice from their medical team about pursuing feeding support, some parents still fear the idea of having their child use a feeding tube. Some worry it will be too difficult to use and that it will draw negative attention or stares to their child, and some feel that by accepting feeding support it is an admission that they have somehow "failed" their child (which is absolutely NOT true!). These are very common feelings among parents and we felt it was important to share one parent's positive experience with transitioning to feeding tube support:

"My son is 3 with CP. He has always eaten and drank orally. Earlier this year, drinking became a long, tough battle. We spent SO MUCH of our time, keeping him hydrated. It was exhausting and stressful. We finally made the decision to get a feeding tube for him. Part of the reasoning was that we wanted to spend our time doing fun things, not trying to get him to eat and drink. It was an extremely tough decision but we are SO THANKFUL that we made the decision! It has been great for him and has freed up so much of our time and has taken a real weight off of my shoulders."

— Alicia Champine

prolonged feeding times, decreased intake, and slow weight gain. Less often, children choke and cough with feedings and are at risk for aspiration, under-nutrition, and breathing problems. If your child has feeding problems, feeding specialists can help you evaluate them. These specialists can include pediatricians, speech pathologists, occupational therapists, nurses, dieticians, gastroenterologists, earn/nose/throat doctors, and others.

Management of Growth, Nutrition, and Feeding Problems

Most management techniques for problems of feeding, growth and nutrition are non-invasive and straightforward. Management is based on assessment of the child's growth and nutritional status and determining whether feeding is efficient and safe. Depending on age and feeding abilities, this may include: mashing, pureeing, thinning or thickening of foods, pacing of feeding, calorie boosts to foods, supplements (e.g. Pediasure, Ensure), seating aids, and special chairs. Physicians can also help manage medical problems that interfere with feeding by prescribing things like oxygen (for chronic lung disease), reflux medicines, and constipation aids.

Despite these management strategies, some children are simply unable to safely take in the needed calories for health and growth. When this happens your medical team will discuss placement of a gastrostomy (also known as a feeding tube or a g-tube). Placement of a gastrostomy is a tool to allow children and families to manage safe feeding and ensure adequate nutrition. Most children with a gastrostomy are able to continue to eat a little bit by mouth (e.g. their favorite treats). For some children the gastrostomy can be used just for liquids (which are often hard to manage safely) and medications, and to serve as "back up" for when children are ill.

IDENTIFY THE SIGNS
The early stages of communication disorders are easier to spot when you know the signs.
For more info visit IdentifyTheSigns.org
American Speech-Language-Hearing Association
Inattentiveness
Buzzing
Failure to Respond
Depression
Isolation
Listening to electronics at High Volumes
Ringing
Muffled Hearing
Frustration
Avoiding Conversation

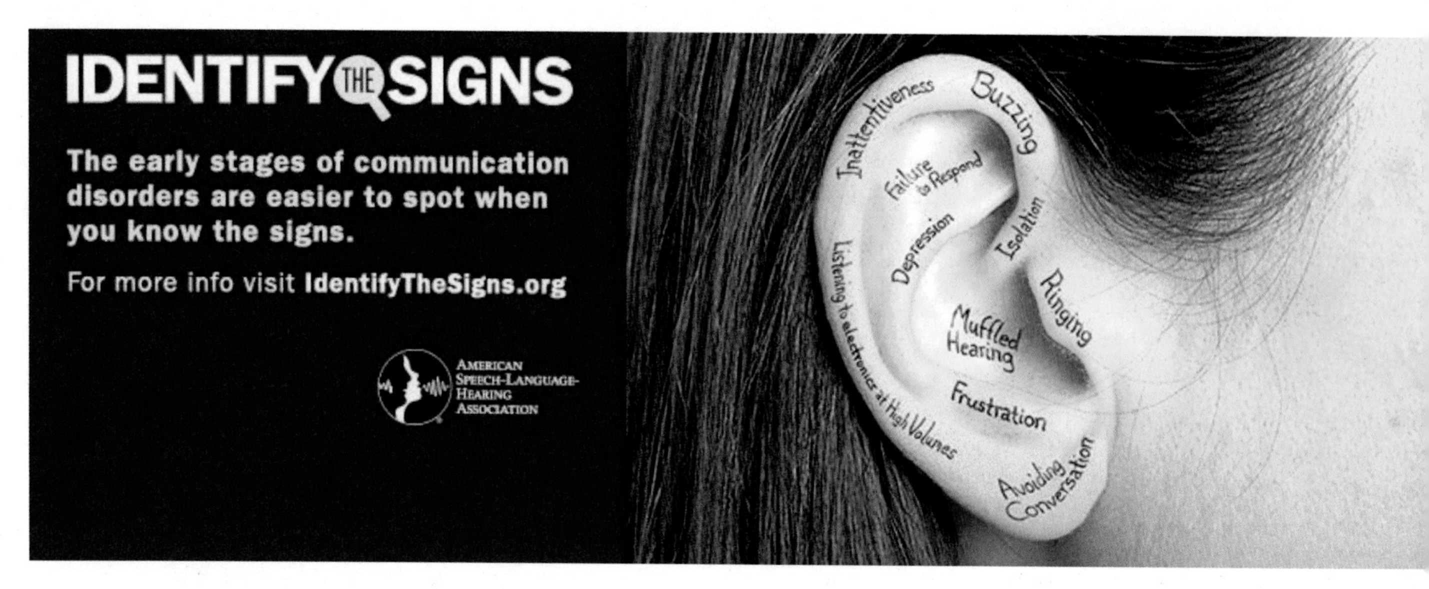

Permission for using graphic granted by the American Speech-Language-Hearing Association.

Communication

HEARING — Research suggests that the most intensive period of speech and language development is during the first three years of life. "If a child is not exposed to language during this period due to hearing loss, he or she will have more difficulty developing spoken or signed language, and reading skills. In addition, during the early stages of life, the brain builds the nerve pathways necessary for understanding auditory information."[10] For these reasons, identifying hearing loss as early as possible enables parents to pursue treatment options to maximize and support the developing child's communication skills.

One Australian study about hearing conducted between 1999 and 2004 included 685 children who had CP. Within this group of participants who had CP 13 percent had some kind of hearing impairment.[11]

Children with CP can have either a conductive or sensorineural hearing loss. It is also possible to have a combination of the two. Conductive hearing loss occurs when sounds are unable to pass from the child's outer ear to their inner ear as the result of a blockage or a disorder of the hearing bones. Sensori-neural hearing loss occurs when there is damage to the sensitive hair cells either inside the cochlea or the auditory nerve.

Identification of new or emerging hearing loss in one or both ears followed by appropriate referral for diagnosis and treatment are the first steps to minimizing their effects on language development and communication.

SPEECH — The risk of a communication disorder increases with cerebral palsy. Speech-language pathologists/therapists (SLP) evaluate communication skills and treat speech and language disorders. This includes both receptive language—what your child is hearing and how they are understanding it—and expressive language—what your child is saying and how they are communicating with others.

The Communication Function Classification System (CFCS) is a measure of current communication skills for someone who has cerebral palsy and other disabilities. It is a five-level system that describes communication in the context of activity and participation levels.

Speech therapists can also evaluate and treat your child for difficulties with motor skills related to eating, drinking and swallowing. The Eating and

IDENTIFY THE SIGNS
The early stages of communication disorders are easier to spot when you know the signs.
For more info visit IdentifyTheSigns.org
American Speech-Language-Hearing Association
Not Understanding or Responding
Unclear Speech
Not Interacting Socially
Not Combining Words
Saying Few Words
Struggling to Talk

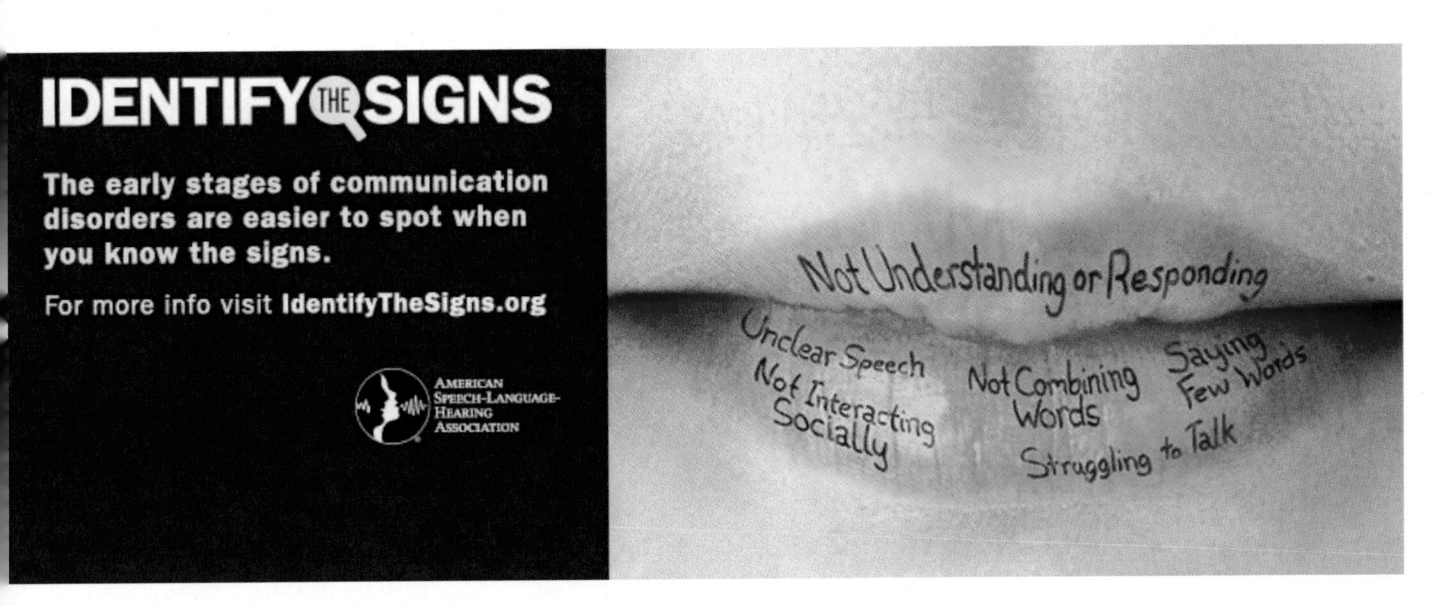

Permission for using graphic granted by the American Speech-Language-Hearing Association.

Drinking Ability Classification System (EDACS) is similar to the evaluations for gross, fine motor, and communications skills in people with CP. It is also a five-level system which provides descriptions of the child's ability to eat and drink.

An annual speech and language screening during birth to 3 years will help determine whether factors such as motor skills, breath support, posture, oral tone and eye gaze are developing fully to support your child's verbal and nonverbal communication. Early intervention may decrease the problems associated with speech and language delays such as:

- Speech that is hard for others to understand
- Difficulty understanding language or expressing language
- Literacy disorders—difficulty reading and writing
- Social-communication disorders—difficulty using verbal and nonverbal language for social purposes

Orthopedics

HIP SURVEILLANCE — Hip surveillance is the process of identifying and monitoring the most important indicators of progressive hip displacement—when the hip socket does not fully cover the top of the thigh bone (femur). **It is important that your child's medical team pay attention to your child's hips as they develop, particularly since pain from hip dislocation has been the number one reported cause of pain in children who have CP.**[12] Although consensus standards of care for hip surveillance in CP have not formally been established in the US, countrywide hip surveillance programs are commonplace in Australia, Sweden, Norway, Finland, Denmark and Scotland. The Australian Academy for Cerebral Palsy and Developmental Medicine (AusACPDM) sees hip surveillance in CP as "an essential part of the strategy for preventing hip displacement and its related problems."

Research demonstrates that the risk of hip subluxation and dislocation is directly related to the individual's mobility and not necessarily the type of CP they have. As severity increases (meaning GMFCS increases) the risk for hip displacement increases. The risk is highest in young children age 2 to 8 years old, then decreases until full growth is reached, usually around 14 to 18 years of age.

The primary measure used in evaluating an x-ray for hip surveillance is called the migration percentage or **Migration Percentage (MP)** or **Migration Index (MI)**. These terms refer to the percentage the head of the hip has moved out of normal alignment. Because the hips change as the child grows, x-rays need to be repeated over time. Each of the national surveillance programs in use throughout the world has slightly different time schedules for getting x-rays. At each radiology visit for hip screening, only a single AP pelvis x-ray should be made to reduce long term radiation exposure.

At this time most orthopedic specialists who treat kids with CP agree on the following: Surgical intervention should be considered for MP>45%; but each case must be assessed individually by an orthopedist experienced in treating children with CP. These specialists can determine the potential risks and benefits of surgical intervention.

GAIT — PROBLEMS WALKING: Children who have CP and begin walking tend to do so later than their same aged peers. Physical therapists are professionals who are able to help them develop their walking skills and offer suggestions for the the best assistive devices to support them along the way, such as a walker or gait trainer. It is not uncommon for children with CP to begin walking on their tip toes and sometimes they may walk with their knees bent or with their legs turning or crossing. These common problems may be very noticeable during the early stages of walking (perhaps at 1-3 years old but it may be later), but may slowly improve over time as the child develops. During this time your child's therapist or medical professional may suggest an evaluation from an orthotist who makes foot braces that may help maintain the alignment of the child's feet and legs.

Another effect of growth is that the bones may become abnormally shaped in response to muscles that do not grow (lengthen) quickly enough. If these problems continue your medical team may suggest surgery to correct these problems. These types of surgeries are typically done by pediatric orthopedic surgeons and usually after the child has had a full evaluation in a special laboratory called a **Gait Analysis Laboratory**. The lab evaluates the child's walking pattern by taking a specialized recording of the activity of the leg muscles as the child walks. These results, along with the doctor's examination, are used to carefully assess and determine the need for surgery. All children and surgeons are different. It may be helpful to seek opinions from more than one experienced specialist.

SCOLIOSIS — SCOLIOSIS IN THE CHILD NOT ABLE TO WALK: Scoliosis means a sideways curvature of the spine causing the child to have increased problems with seating and head control. In more severe cases, problems with increased pain and breathing may interfere with how well some of the internal organs function. Severe scoliosis occurs commonly in children who are not able to sit by themselves or hold their head up. It is less common in children who are able to move independently.

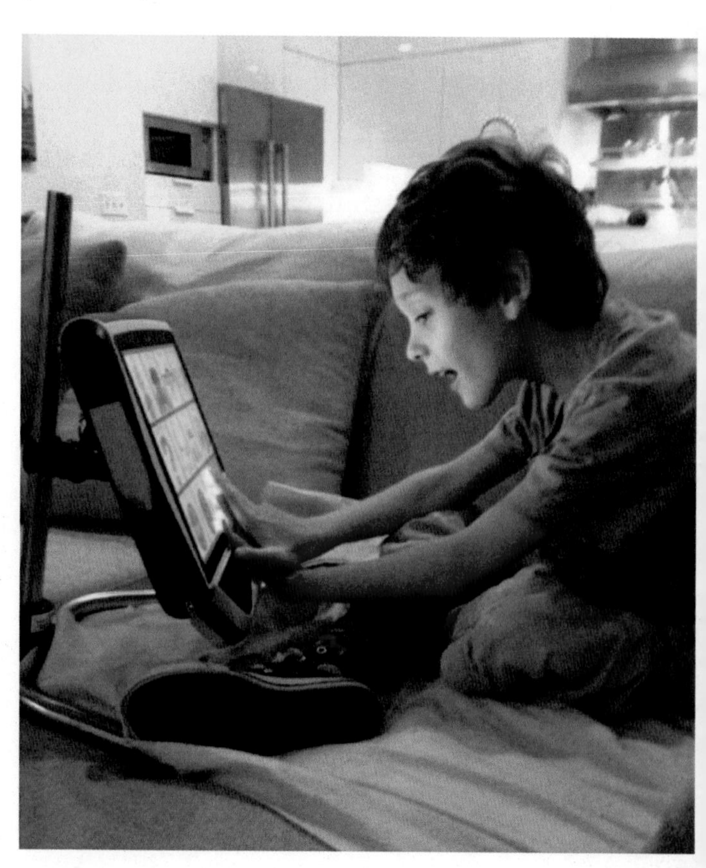

Some children are given body braces to stop the progression of scoliosis. Although some of these braces may help the child to sit better and are useful for this purpose, it is not uncommon that consistent bracing is not enough to prevent the progression of scoliosis. At some point a spinal fusion, a surgery performed by an orthopedic surgeon, may be proposed to address the worsening scoliosis.

Learning/Cognition

Childhood is not a race to see how quickly a child can read, write and count. Childhood is a small window of time to learn and develop at the pace which is right for each individual child. Earlier is not better."

Magda Gerber, Early Childhood Educator

NEUROPSYCHOLOGY ASSESSMENTS — **A Neuropsychological assessment is used to identify how cerebral palsy has disrupted your child's cognitive/behavioral functioning.** This type of screening will evaluate your child's capabilities in multiple settings (home, school, community). It can identify strengths and weaknesses that may impact how your child interprets and approaches circumstances throughout the day, or how your child functions in school. Your pediatrician may refer your child to a neuropsychologist, or your child's early education or early intervention team may work with one.

During this assessment, a trained neuropsychologist should take special care to ensure you child's abilities are assessed in a fair and valid manner. They will take into account the impact that seating, positioning, breath support, level of fatigue, visual impairment, etc., can have upon your child's ability to complete standardized tests. Moreover, testing be conducted using your child's preferred/best method of responding (pointing, single word responses, eye-gaze, sip-and-puff, augmented communication device, etc.). Accommodations for testing often include shortening the length of testing, reducing/eliminating articulation and motor requirements, integration of assistive technology, and presenting more difficult tasks in the morning when children are more rested.

There is not a generic "neuropsychological profile" of children with CP, as skills and abilities can range from normal to impaired. There are trends, however, to suggest that children with CP often have non-verbal reasoning deficits, reduced overall cognitive abilities, difficulties with attention, and impairments in visuospatial/visuoperceptual skills. While it is important for neuropsychologists to identify areas of deficit and impairment to justify treatment and funding, it is also very important that the assessment identify adaptive and/or cognitive skill gains as well as emerging strengths and capabilities.

SENSORY INTEGRATION — The senses work together continuously sending and receiving information to and from the brain and nervous system. This sensory feedback system helps the individual understand themselves and their relationship to their environment. When there are problems with sensory integration it means the brain has problems interpreting and organizing the information coming from the senses. This can create confusion, discomfort and learning difficulties for the individual (as mentioned in the section above). For people with CP any one of the senses can be affected and these impairments may affect each child differently.

The five senses most of us are familiar with are:

- VISION — visual perception
- HEARING — auditory perception
- TOUCH — tactile perception
- SMELL — olfactory perception
- TASTE — oral perception

Two senses we may not be familiar with are:

- VESTIBULAR SENSE — the perception of balance and spatial orientation for the purpose of coordinating movement
- PROPRIOCEPTIVE SENSE — the perception of where parts of the body are in relationship to one another and in space. As an example, even if a person closes their eyes they should be able to know if their arm is by their side or up in the air.

An individual with cerebral palsy often has difficulty using sensory information to determine when, where and how to move. This can cause problems with postural control, postural reactions, balance, eye-hand coordination, and the ability to make goal-directed movements. Sensory integration therapy aims to help the individual better organize, understand and respond to incoming sensory information from the environment and their body.[13]

The Council on Children with Disabilities of the American Academy of Pediatrics (AAP) released a statement entitled "Sensory integration therapies for children with developmental and behavioral disorders."[14] The Council acknowledged that there is no universally accepted framework for the diagnosis of sensory processing disorder and that evidence for the efficacy of sensory-based therapies is limited; but it advised that occupational therapy with the use of sensory-based therapies may be acceptable as one component of a comprehensive treatment plan.

Oral Health

Tooth decay issues are prevalent for people with CP and arise for a variety of reasons. Regular check-ups address oral health issues such as tooth decay, tooth grinding and reflux (which may require follow-up with a specialist). Because of difficulty chewing and swallowing some people with CP may eat starchy food which can contribute to increased tooth decay. Some may take medications or may breathe more through their mouth which can cause their mouths to dry out. This can mean less saliva to wash out remaining food particles and bacteria in the mouth. Further, it may be difficult in some cases to access and brush their back teeth.

Reflux, tooth grinding, and TMJ or jaw dysfunctions are painful and can wear away enamel. This makes the teeth more vulnerable to cavities.

Challenges to maintaining dental health in CP (ie; removing decay and filling cavities):

- Oral hypersensitivity.
- Positioning.
- Hyper or hypo active gag reflex. Having a hyper or hypo active gag reflex can also make it difficult to remove fluids or to cough to clear fluids.
- Bite reflexes can make it hard to brush teeth.

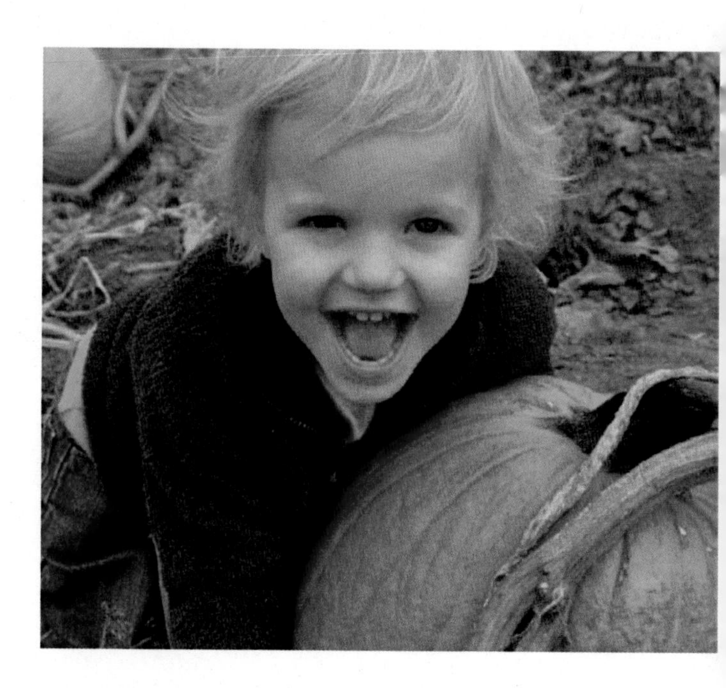

Products and strategies to help dental hygiene for people w/ CP:

- Toothpastes that are gels are more water-soluble. They may be tolerated better and work better because they clear out of the mouth easier. Watch for fluoride intake especially in younger children or those prone to swallowing toothpaste since there are guidelines for how much fluoride can be safely ingested (See the American Dental Association website for more information.)
- Consider brushes with a rotating head, wide handle, brushes modified with a tennis ball on the end so that it is easier to hold.
- Rinsing to remove debris is one of the most important strategies in maintaining oral health.
- Brush and floss as much as possible to maintain a more neutral PH in the mouth; a more acidic oral PH leads to increased susceptibility to dental decay and cavities.
- Use a dry mouth spray (ask your dental care provider for recommendations).
- Use a fluoride varnish—consult with your dentist to see if this is appropriate.

Pain Management

It is critical that pediatricians be aware that chronic pain often begins in childhood for people with CP. Pain in CP is often underrecognized and undertreated and it may have multiple causes. Identifying its source can be complex. In some cases, doctors and caregivers may attribute pain to the underlying spasticity and contractures, when in fact, it may be due to an undetected, treatable problem (i.e urinary tract infection).

Parents are encouraged to ask their child's pediatricians and other professionals about addressing pain. In cases where communication with the child is difficult, a parent acts as a critical liaison between the clinician and patient. Partner with your child's doctors to try to identify where your child may be experiencing pain so that the doctor may work on treating its underlying causes.

In 2013 Dr. Darcy Fehlings of the University of Toronto led researchers at Holland Bloorview Kids Rehabilitation Hospital in a study about pain in children with CP. **They discovered that more than 25 percent of children with CP seen by physicians have moderate to severe chronic pain limiting their activity, and that more than half of participants were in some kind of pain that was not being treated.**[15] This study demonstrated that hip pain and increased muscle tone are common causes of pain for children. It is particularly important for clinicians to look for pain in people who have dyskinetic forms of CP that include dystonia. Pain due to dystonia is often overlooked, yet it is the second most common cause of pain for people who have CP. Hip dislocation is number one.

Developing a strategy to prevent, assess, and manage chronic pain for kids with CP is key to improving their health and quality of life.

Underdiagnosed causes of pain in CP include: Dystonia, gastro-intestinal problems, hypertonia, tooth decay, constipation, reflux, and hip subluxation (see the section above on "hip surveillance").

Factors contributing to sleep disturbances in CP can generally be categorized into eight areas:

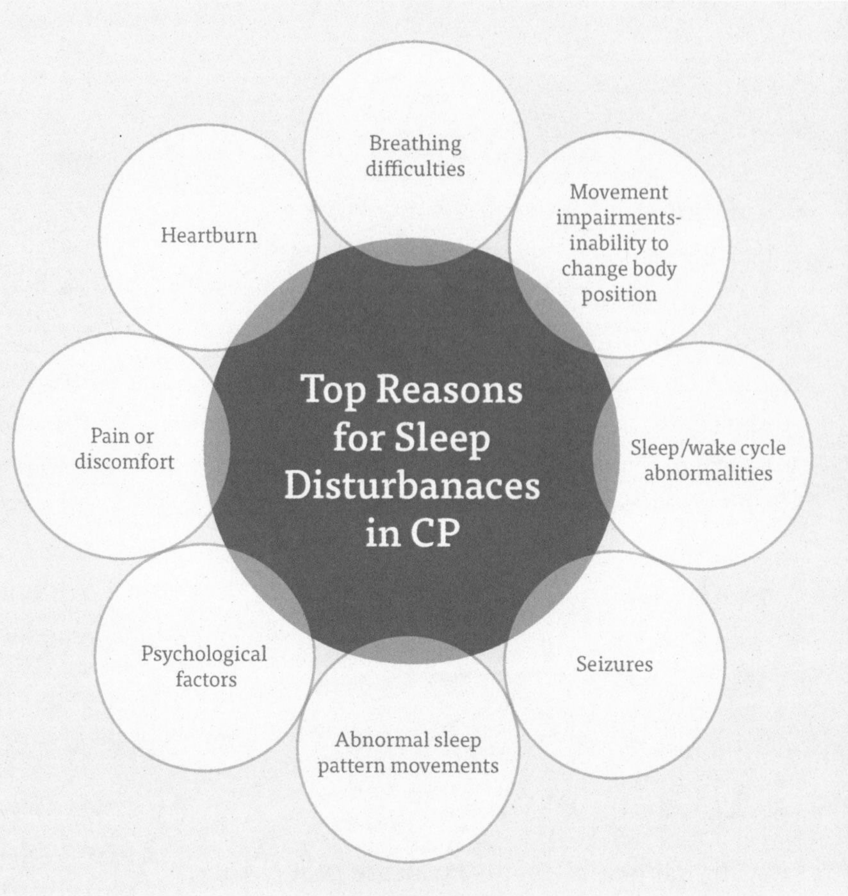

Potential Consequences of Bladder Dysfunction

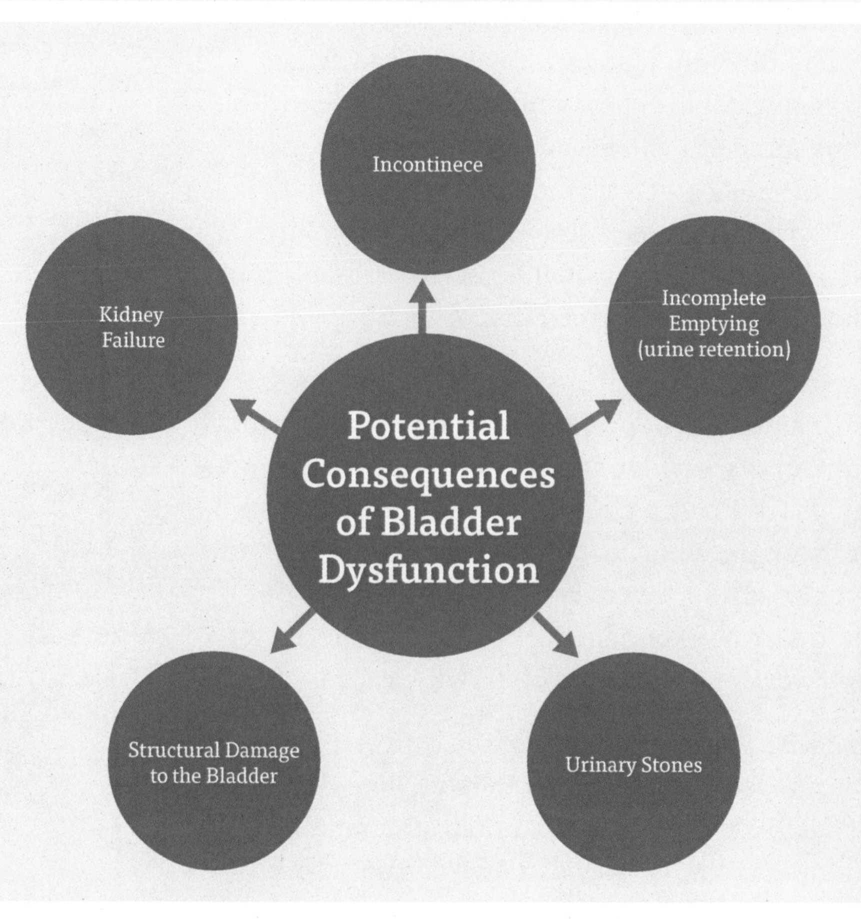

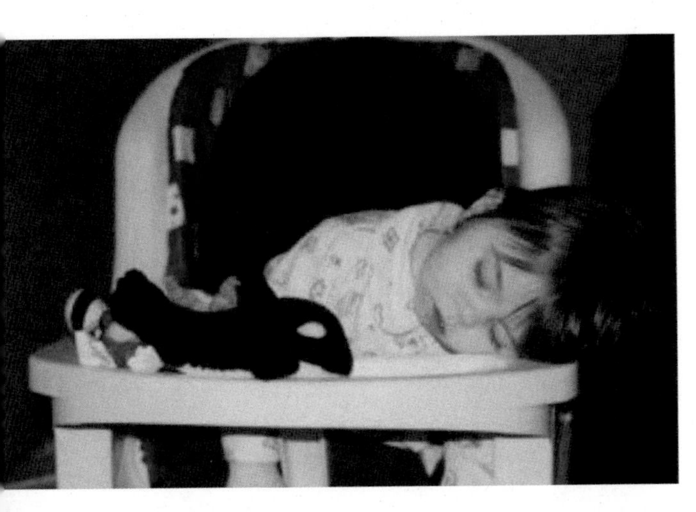

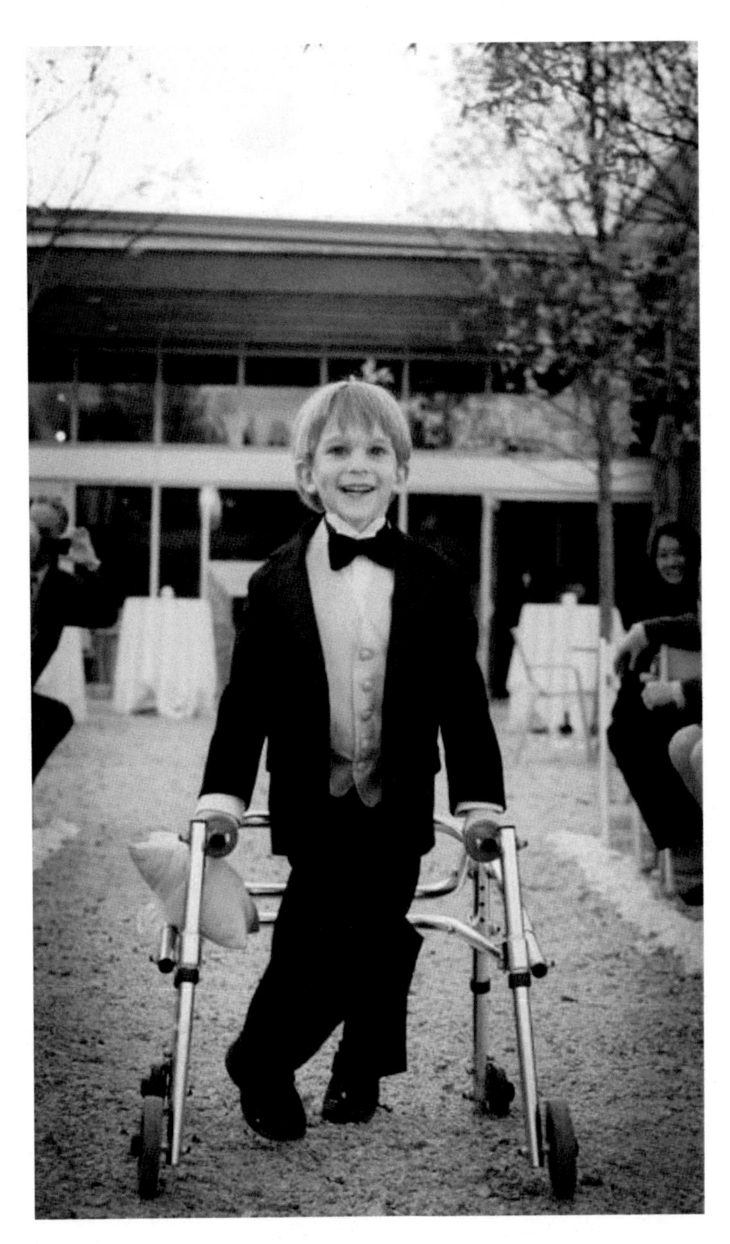

Sleep Disorders

Sleep issues in the general population are very common throughout infancy, childhood, and preadolescence. Studies estimate that sleep disturbances vary from 5% to 40% among all children.[16–18] In children with CP it is important to investigate and address sleep disturbances because of their potential persistence and severity. Sleep disturbances may also lead to difficulties with the child's cognition and behavior during the day, as well as affect parents and the energy they may have to care for their child.[19]

Urodynamics

Up to 70-80% of the CP population has problems with urine control or bladder overactivity.[20] Doctors and family members often consider urinary assessments less important in people with CP because incontinence is seen as a quality of life issue rather than a health concern. Also, lack of urine control may be quickly attributed to diminished cognition or failure to achieve age specific continence milestones without considering potential underlying dysfunction of the urinary tract.

Urodynamic testing is a procedure that evaluates how well an individual can store urine and empty their bladder. This test is usually performed by a urologist and involves the bladder being filled and emptied through a small catheter. The volumes, pressure within the bladder and urine flow are all recorded. Often the study is done in conjunction with radiologic imaging to provide maximum information about how the bladder is functioning.

Addressing urinary tract problems as soon as they begin can improve outcomes and possibilities for preventing increasing problems in the urinary tract which are shared in the diagram to the right:

Approaches available for treating bladder dysfunction in the CP population include pharmacological, catheterization and biofeedback techniques. Talk to your doctor if you have concerns about your child's urinary tract function.

Vision

Children with CP are at risk for various kinds of problems with their vision. There may be problems related to the structures of the eye and how it is working (i.e focusing) called **ocular impairments**. There may also be problems with the visual pathways and the areas of the brain that receive and make sense of incoming visual information from the eyes. This is commonly referred to as **cortical visual impairment (CVI)**. Vision is a complex area of development that has a tremendous impact on the child's ability to learn. Some can be treated effectively over time, or vision support services can be implemented to ensure the child may effectively access their environment.

There are many different types of vision professionals listed below who can provide evaluations and support for vision impairments. Ask your child's primary care doctor, rehabilitation physician, or developmental pediatrician for guidance about which professionals to contact for services. In some areas you may not have all of these specialists and will need to work with your medical team to determine who can best address your concerns or provide the appropriate vision services.

Medical professionals and optometrists diagnose vision problems:

NEURO OPHTHALMOLOGIST — An MD who completes at least 5 years of clinical training after medical school. They are usually board certified in neurology, ophthalmology, or both and have received specialized training and expertise in problems of the eye, brain, nerves and muscles. Almost half of the brain is used for vision-related activities, including sight and moving the eyes. Neuro-ophthalmologists treat eye disorders and visual disorders that occur in the brain rather than the eyes themselves.

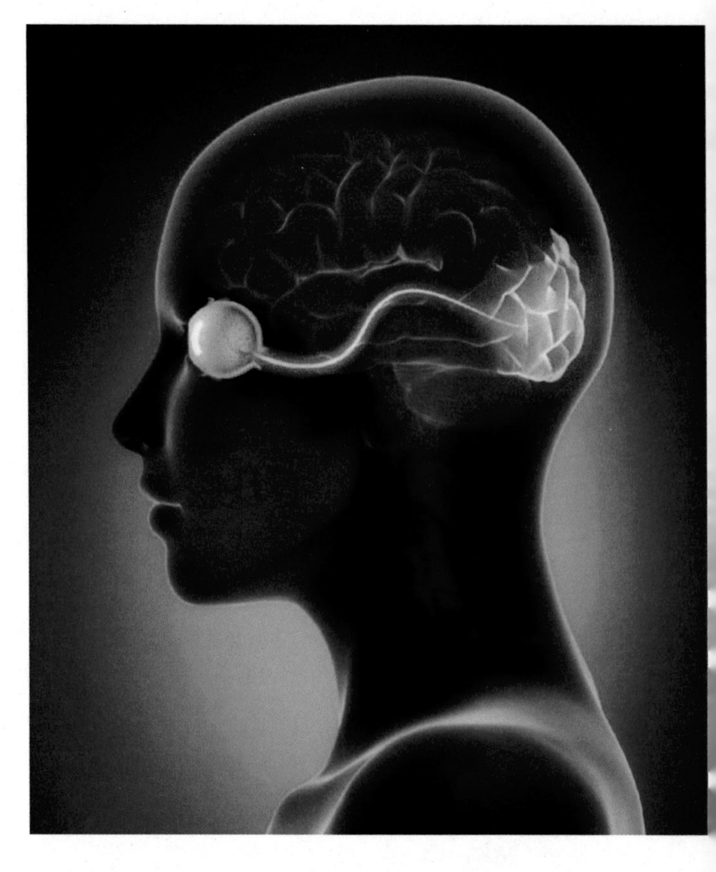

OPHTHALMOLOGIST — An MD who is trained to diagnose and treat disorders of the eye and optic nerve. They treat with surgery, lenses, medicines or certain therapeutic interventions such as patching for strabismus.

OPTOMETRIST — An optometrist receives a doctor of optometry (OD) degree after completing four years of optometry school, preceded by three or more years of college. Optometrists are licensed to perform eye exams and vision tests, prescribe and dispense corrective lenses, and detect certain eye abnormalities.

OPTICIAN — An optician is trained to design, verify and fit eyeglass lenses and frames, contact lenses, and other devices to correct eyesight. Opticians are not permitted to diagnose or treat eye diseases.

LOW VISION SPECIALIST — An optometrist who specializes in the needs of individuals who are visually impaired and thus, require specialized lenses and magnifying equipment.

Vision specialists who provide classroom support:

TEACHER OF THE VISUALLY IMPAIRED — A teacher who usually has a Master's degree in providing educational services to children with ocular and cortical forms of visual impairment.

ORIENTATION & MOBILITY SPECIALIST — A professional who has certification in teaching techniques to assist visually impaired and blind individuals to be properly oriented in space and to move safely through the environment.

Both of these specialists conduct vision evaluations and educational assessments to determine how the child is using their vision and how they can best be supported in the classroom. These functional vision assessments are categorized into those used for children with ocular disorders and those for children with cortical visual impairment, such as the CVI Range. The CVI Range developed by Dr. Roman-Lantzy is explained in depth in the book *Cortical Visual Impairment: An Approach to Assessment and Intervention*.

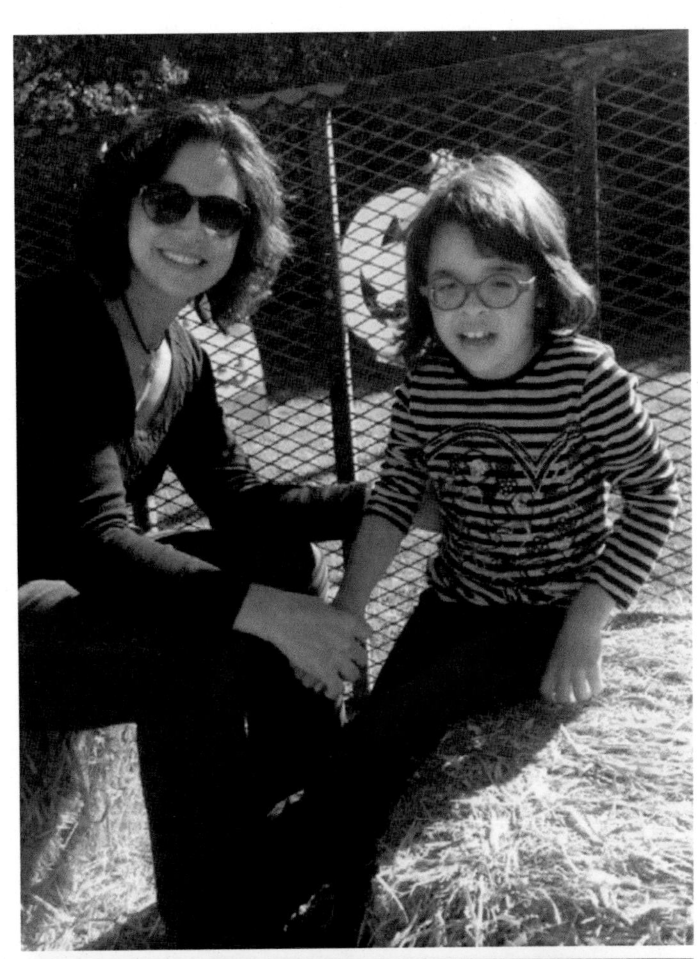

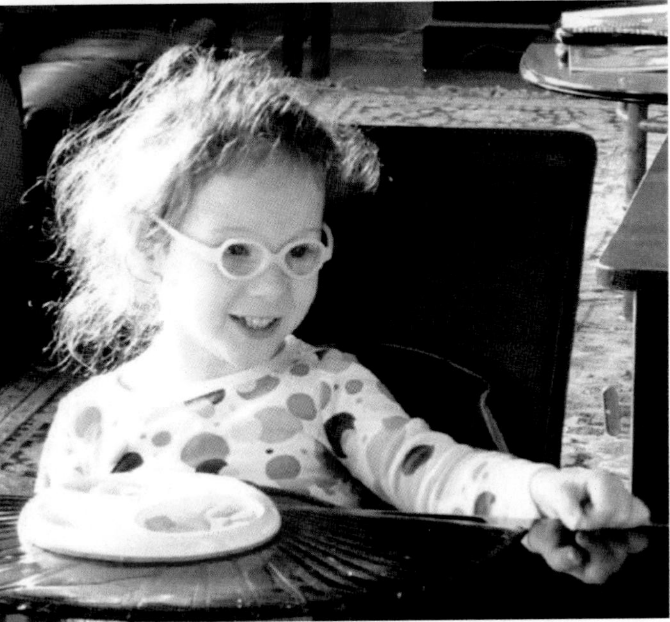

AN IMPORTANT NOTE REGARDING CORTICAL VISUAL IMPAIRMENT (CVI):

CVI is the leading cause of pediatric visual impairment in developed nations.[21-22] Since people with CP have had some type of neurological disturbance, it is possible that the areas of the brain associated with visual processing may have also been affected. CVI may be present in children who do not have ocular impairments and who have had a normal eye exam. This condition is diagnosed using different techniques that may lead to inconsistent results. For this reason it is critical for parents to follow their instincts if they believe their child is not visually attending to objects, people, or environments. Specialized assessments and interventions can facilitate improvements in visual processing and their functional vision—the child's ability to use their vision in everyday life.

SECTION 6

You, Your Family & CP

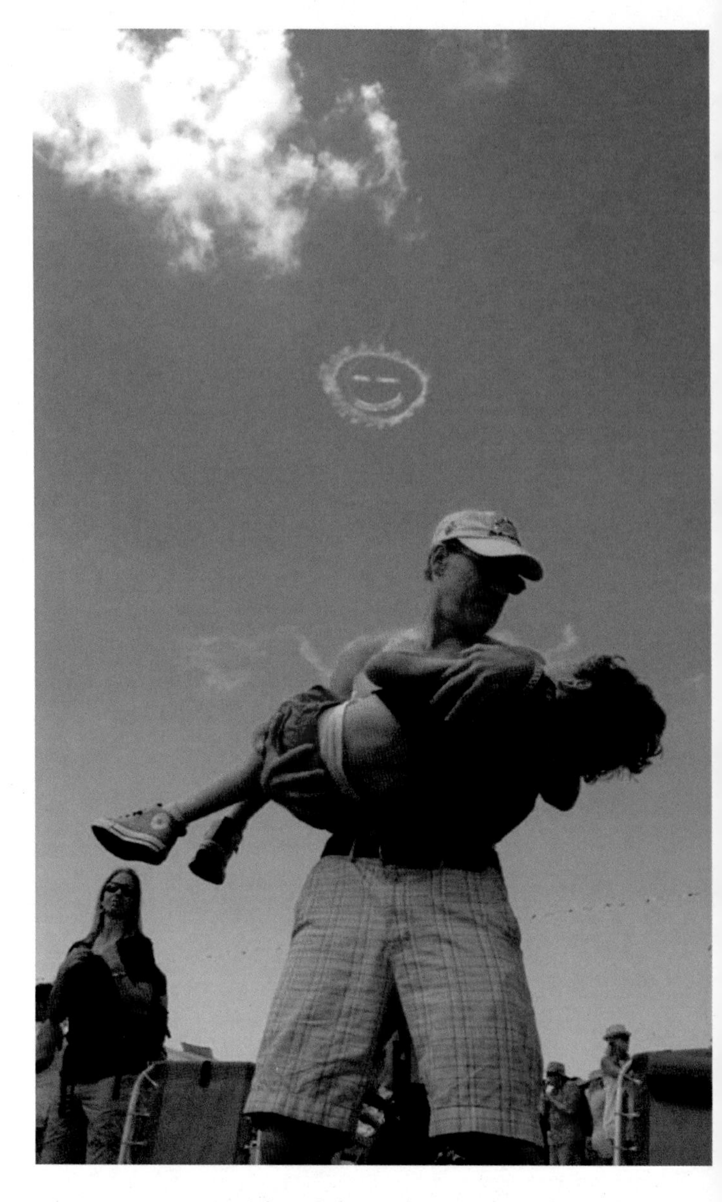

Sharing the diagnosis with family and friends

AFTER YOU LEARN THAT YOUR CHILD HAS CP, it can be difficult to share this information with family members and friends. You may feel concerned about how people close to you will treat you and your child. Although you cannot control the reactions of your family and friends, you can educate them and provide guidance about how you would like them to treat your child and family. You may find it helpful to ask them what they understand about cerebral palsy and clear up any misunderstanding they may have about the condition. If you do not feel comfortable discussing the diagnosis in depth, you may direct people to a reliable source of information about CP like this Tool Kit. There are other resources that may also be helpful in the "Additional Resources" section of the Tool Kit.

Once you have shared this information, you may feel sad or angry about the way people react to you or your child. Keep in mind that people often do not understand or know what to say to be supportive. It's sometimes difficult to be patient in these circumstances. Your family may need time to learn, adjust and work through their own feelings. They may need opportunities to get to know your child as a person outside of their diagnosis of cerebral palsy. You can also help shape the perspectives of people close to you by emphasizing your child's strengths and by being direct about the ways in which you and your child may need support.

Take the initiative and discuss your child's condition with family and friends, explaining how to approach, talk to, play with, and care for your child. You can introduce the topic of your child's diagnosis directly (which may be easier in the long run) or bring information and expectations more naturally into a conversation as circumstances arise. Set aside dedicated time to speak with people individually.

If you are troubled by the assumptions people are making about your child or the terms they are using to describe them, you can either model your preferred response, or tell them how you feel. Modeling means repeating what has been said to you, but replacing the words of your choice for the words you disliked in the original comment. The more you talk about your child having cerebral palsy, the more you will learn about how you wish to handle these conversations. You may even wish to talk about or rehearse these kinds of conversations with your spouse, relative or close friend.

Examples of *Teachable Moments*

I knew someone who had cerebral palsy who went to school but I was surprised she was capable of learning."

RESPONSE: "Many people assume that all people with CP have the same difficulties but that is not the case. Some people with CP have intellectual disabilities and others don't. Also, having an intellectual (or physical) disability does not mean someone cannot attend school and learn alongside their peers.

It's a good thing John can't understand anything I am saying."

RESPONSE: "Actually, John can understand everything you are saying. Even though he is not able to communicate to you with words, he can hear and understand you perfectly."

"My friend's son is retarded too."

Before answering some of you may need to take a breath and consider that this person is probably just trying to identify with your experience (even if it is in a remote way) rather than trying to offend you. You could say a number of things here to replace the "R-word" including "special needs", "disability", or simply say that your child "needs extra support." Some people may also wish to more openly express their feelings about the "R-word", the assumptions it conveys and why it upsets them. Keep in mind that although this term has very negative connotations, it started out as a formal medical description and many people use it innocently to mean "disability." Not all people (especially older generations) mean to be offensive.

RESPONSE: "I'm not exactly sure what you mean when you use that word. Shari has some extra needs but she is a lot like any other child."

The following is a great blog post called "Rebel Muscles" about how to describe CP. It was written by popular special needs blogger Ellen Seidman who shares her stories and insights at *Love that Max*.

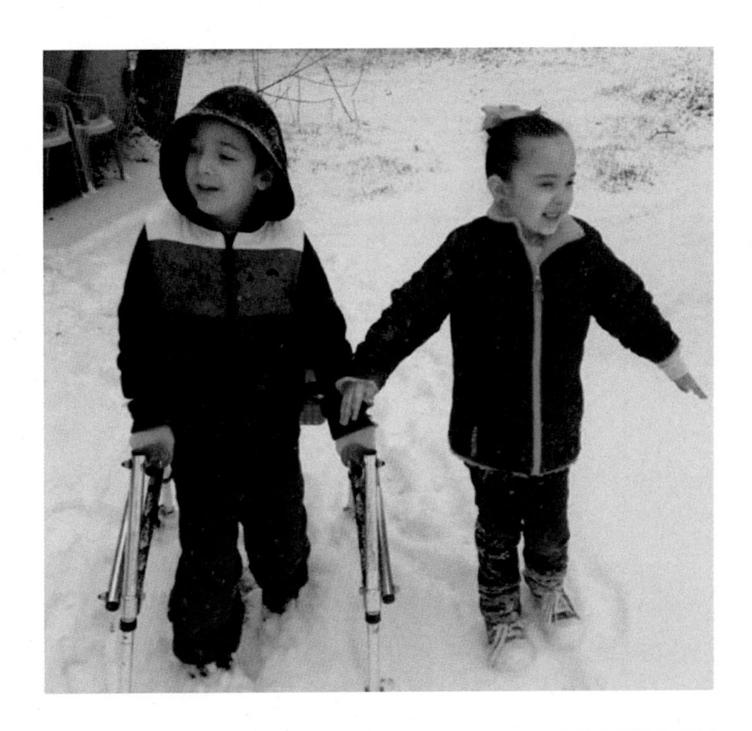

What a parent of a child with special needs wishes her friends knew:

1. We feel alone sometimes. Please don't intentionally or unintentionally exclude us or our children from activities with your children. Your children may be the only children that they can learn to develop friendships with. If a social situation doesn't seem appropriate for our child, leave it to us to decide whether to attend or not.
2. Please don't feel uncomfortable around our family because you don't understand. Half the time we don't understand either, but we need the sense of normalness that your friendship provides.
3. Let your children ask questions. It's totally ok with us. We love answering and educating your children about how our child isn't any different from yours.
4. Sometimes we feel like venting about things we know you don't understand. And it's ok if you don't know what to say. Just being a friend with an ear is all we need at times.
5. Our parenting situation isn't all that different from yours. It's still parenting and it's still kids, we just have some extra things attached to our lifestyle.
6. Even though our lives may seem impossible at times (trust me we feel that way too!) we are very happy. Our special child has taught us so much about life, happiness and really appreciating the small miracles of everyday things. It actually makes us feel pretty damn lucky that we get to deeply appreciate what others take for granted.
7. We get jealous. Yes I'll admit that when I see a 1 year old say or do something my 6 year old can't do or say it sucks! But when my 6 year old still does the sweet wonderful things that a typical child has long ago stopped doing, such as cuddling, petting my hair and looking at me with the most adoring eyes, it makes me appreciate my life anew every single day.

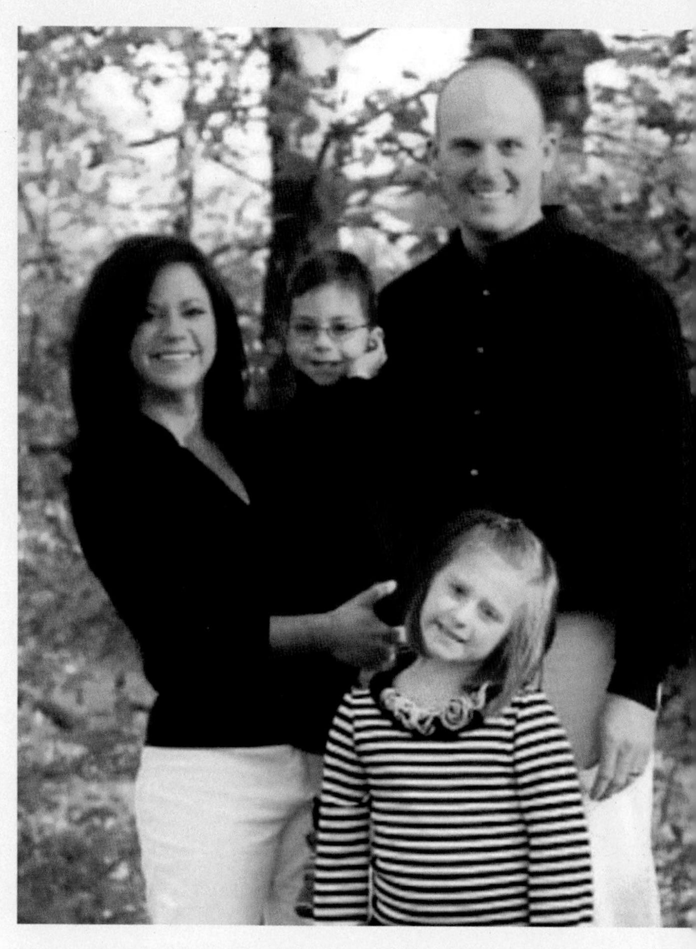

The Combs have been married for 10 years and have two children. Their son was born at 32 weeks and has a diagnosis of Cerebral Palsy, Hydrocephalus, and Epilepsy.

8. We are tired. And if I may not join in the monthly girls nights out, or miss a few social happenings it doesn't mean I'm being a bad friend. It just means I may need some down time, or we have so much going on with therapies, doctors, appointments etc. But please don't give up on us. We still love you and still need your friendship.
9. We worry. We worry all the time—about doctors, school, the future. And it's ok. We know our future is yet to reveal itself, it's all wait and see. And we know you know that too, and it's ok to talk about it.

Pitfalls of Predictions

As your child develops you are likely to get predictions about their future. For example, you may hear statements such as "Bobby will never walk" or "Bobby should be able to walk." Be wary of any specific predictions about your child's future abilities because CP presents uniquely in each individual. This uniqueness means that accurate predictions are hard to make.

Although you may see similarities among children with cerebral palsy, you cannot base your child's developmental timeline or particular support needs on the development of another child with cerebral palsy. Sometimes parents are given the worst prognosis and their children go on to develop better than anyone could have imagined. Alternatively, doctors may offer a more optimistic prognosis and the child's development does not unfold as the physician had thought. This can leave a parent feeling guilty and wondering what they may have done to prevent their child from reaching the potential the doctor envisioned.

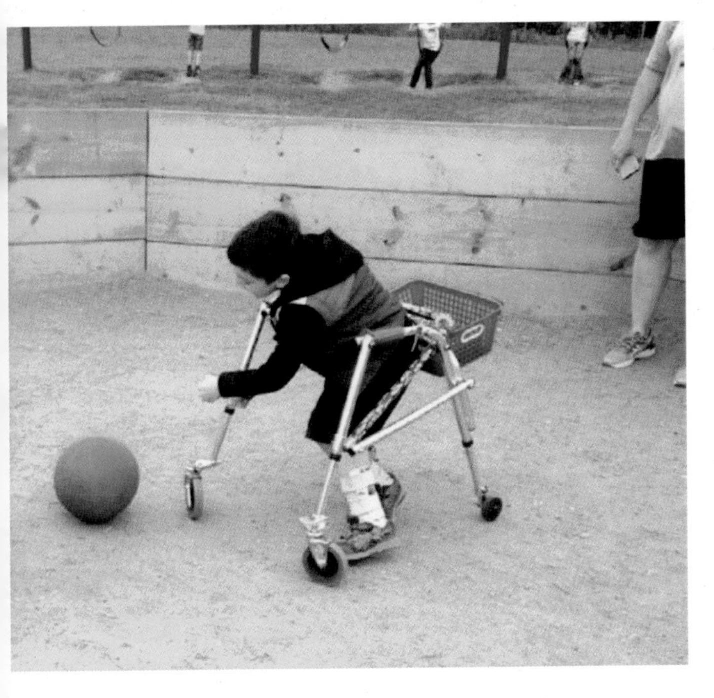

"There is no 'box,' no 'one size fits all' for cerebral palsy. There are common symptoms and conditions that may accompany CP but the future abilities of your child cannot be known, nor the time frames in which developmental milestones will be met. I would encourage you, as the parent/caregiver, to focus on your child in the now and how to help them build on emerging skills. Remember that your child's developmental time frame is their own. Comparing your child to another is like comparing apples to oranges."

Christina Youngblood, Parent of Devin, Age 6

Finding a healthy state of mind between remaining open to positive change and being realistic about what you may expect for your child is difficult but critical. What you can do is make the commitment to address your child's present needs for support and to lead them to whatever their greatest potential may be.

Impact of a CP Diagnosis on Family

Family counseling

CP affects the whole family. Family members may feel confused, jealous, guilty, angry, sad, and fearful. Coming to terms with the emotions brought on by a CP diagnosis can be very challenging, even for the most mentally and emotionally healthy person.

Make sure you have the support you need during this challenging time. You may benefit from counseling individually, as a couple, or as a family. For some of you this may be your first time feeling that you need some assistance working through your feelings or problems. There is no shame in seeking help. As the parent or caregiver you have to ensure you maintain your emotional, physical, mental, and spiritual health. The better care you take of yourself, the more energy and strength you will have for your child.

One last thing that can be of help to the single parent, is to **establish routine**. Having a set routine is not only good for you but good for your child as well. Having a set time for things such as dinner, baths, etc...can help decrease stress levels because you and your child know what's next. You know that by a certain time that you will be done for the day in the care of your child and it gives you something to look forward to, as well as time to de-stress and reflect on the day. Overall, no matter how you became a single parent, one must remember that at the end of the day the word single does not matter, it is the word Parent that matters. You will always be a parent first.

Take care of yourself!
You can't pour from an empty cup.

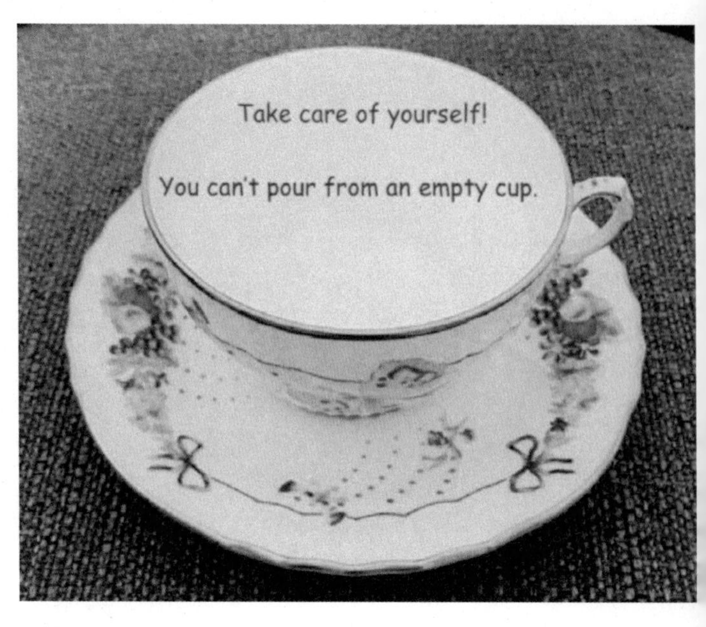

Sibling support

The impact of having a sibling with a disability varies depending on the individual, their personality and developmental age. For many, the experience is a positive, enriching one that teaches them to accept other people as they are. Others may experience bitterness and resentment towards their parents or their affected sibling. They may feel jealous, neglected, or rejected as they observe their parents' attention and energy more focused on the child with special needs. It also is common for siblings to swing back and forth between feeling positive and negative emotions. It's important to take time to talk openly with your children about their sibling who has CP and explain the condition as best you can in terms the child can relate to. They may need professional help processing these big feelings and their conflicting emotions of both loving their sibling and perhaps also feeling annoyed or resentful of them and their disability.

Parents often report that no matter what issues siblings may have at home with their brother or sister with special needs, outside of the home they are typically very loyal to their sibling and do their best to defend and protect them. The experience and knowledge gained by having a sibling with special needs also seems to make children more

Single Parenting Needs

by Cheryl Major, Mother of Monty, age 13

Being a single parent of a special needs child, specifically of a child with CP, can be a challenging yet rewarding task. Upon your child's diagnosis, you are given the resources that will help support your child such as therapies, doctors, equipment vendors etc... but what about you? Where's your support? What about resources for you? Not only are you a parent of a child with cerebral palsy, but you are a single parent. It is easy to give into feelings of self pity but eventually you must come around to accepting your circumstances and knowing that you have to work a little bit harder at meeting the needs of your child.

Despite the circumstances of how you ended up on the journey of single parenthood, it is important to remember that you are very much capable of parenting a child that has different needs from those of their typical peers. **You are not alone in this journey.** A lot of single parents find it hard to reach out to others, fearing that no one will understand what they are going through as a single parent of a special needs child or fear that they may be judged because they are single. **Reaching out for support, not only makes you feel less alone, but it may also help you form new relationships with others who are in a similar situation as you.**

In some children with CP, lifting is required and, as a single parent, you will often find yourself lifting your child alone. **Exercising, lifting small weights, and doing some simple yoga poses can help maintain your body so that you'll be able to help your child. Eating healthy is also very important for a parent to keep their energy up in order to care for their child with CP. It can be very easy for one to just grab a quick high calorie snack or hit the nearest drive-thru between doctors' appointments.** Remember being a single parent of a child with CP can be physically and mentally draining and you need proper nutrients in order to maintain your body. One must also keep in mind that your child could also fall into your bad eating habits as well so it's best to keep a supply of healthy foods in your home at all times.

Having good respite care can help parents get time for themselves. Respite care is a service that provides a break for parents of children with special healthcare needs by providing a trained person to come and stay with your child while you do things such as go to lunch or simply go upstairs and take a nap.

accepting and appreciative of differences. They tend to be more aware of the difficulties others may be going through, and often surprise adults with their wisdom, insight and empathy.[23] SibShops and ForeverSibs are two national resources offering programs for siblings of people with CP and other conditions. Sibshops offers local programming throughout the US and ForeverSibs offers support by mail.

Respite Care and Resources

Respite care is a service that provides temporary relief, be it overnight or for an hour, to the caregiver(s) of a child with a disability. For a parent/guardian caring for a child with CP can be physically and mentally exhausting. This service allows for a registered caregiver, or in some states a family member, to come into your home and care for the child with CP. Respite care offers a great opportunity for families to get a full night's rest, couples date night, or whatever you may need to recharge. Taking advantage of this service does not imply that you are unable to care for your child's needs. It means that you recognize, that in order to continue caring for your child, you must keep yourself healthy and rested. The amount of respite care hours vary depending on the state in which you live and, in some instances, what your medical insurance provider allows.

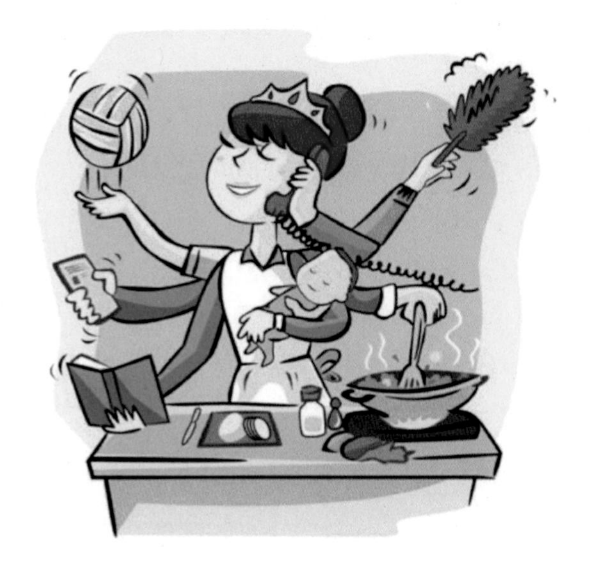

Reaching Out for Help

An excerpt from parent blogger Alisa Bentley

"At first, I was skeptical to let a stranger into my home to help me with things that I can do on my own for my daughter. Then, I started talking to parents that have a personal care assistant for their child with special needs, all with varying levels of assistance needed. I liked what I was hearing and decided to talk to a provider. I even went as far as filling out the paperwork. That was in May, and it sat in my "To Do Basket" for almost a month before I pulled it out and sent my husband to submit the application in person. A month later (last week) I received a phone call that our daughter had been assigned a caseworker to review our request for services. I hung up the phone, sat on the couch and cried. **I needed help, and admitting this to myself was so overwhelming.**

When the caseworker arrived she asked all the standard questions that I have become accustomed to over the years. I ran around after my daughter while answering her questions, keeping it "professional" so no information would be missed. At the very end, as we were wrapping up and my daughter began watching a Barney music video, the caseworker asked "is there anything else you would like to tell me about your daughter or your family that will help us determine what services you would benefit from?" **Oh brother, here it comes... big crocodile tears! I wanted to tell her how we are doing great and keeping it all together, but a little extra help would be appreciated.** I wanted to tell her that having someone come into our home a couple hours a week would allow me to take care of my household responsibilities while my daughter still receives one on one attention. I wanted to tell her how helpful her big brother is, but I didn't want to keep putting more expectations on him. I wanted to tell her how proud we are of our children and what our family has overcome. **Instead, with tears streaming down my face, I simply asked her for help. Our journey is going to be a long one, and in order for me to be the best Mom I can be to my children, I need to ask *and* accept help when possible."** The caseworker gave me a hug, told me I was doing a great job with both of my children, and said that she would be in touch soon.

SECTION 7

Early Intervention & Early Education

What is Early Intervention?

EARLY INTERVENTION (EI) PROVIDES SUPPORTIVE SERVICES for infants and toddlers between birth and three years who meet their state's criteria for a developmental delay or who have been diagnosed with physical or mental conditions with high probabilities of resulting in developmental delays.

Early Intervention services are offered through a public or private agency and are provided in different settings, such as your home, a clinic, a neighborhood daycare center or Head Start program, a hospital, or your local health department. **Initial evaluation and assessment of your child will be provided free of charge.** Additional services may also be provided at no cost, although this may vary from state to state. Some states charge a "sliding-scale" fee for services.

Eligibility for EI is determined after a child has been evaluated by a health professional. Some children are diagnosed at birth with a condition that makes them eligible for EI, while other children may not be evaluated until they have a documented delay in reaching milestones. Parents can get a referral for Early Intervention services through their health care provider or they can contact their local EI program directly and ask for an evaluation.

You can find your EI office and state eligibility requirements here.

What Services are Offered Through EI?
Through Early Intervention service providers and families work together to develop customized plans to help build and maximize the child's skills as early as possible. Services provided by Early Intervention include:

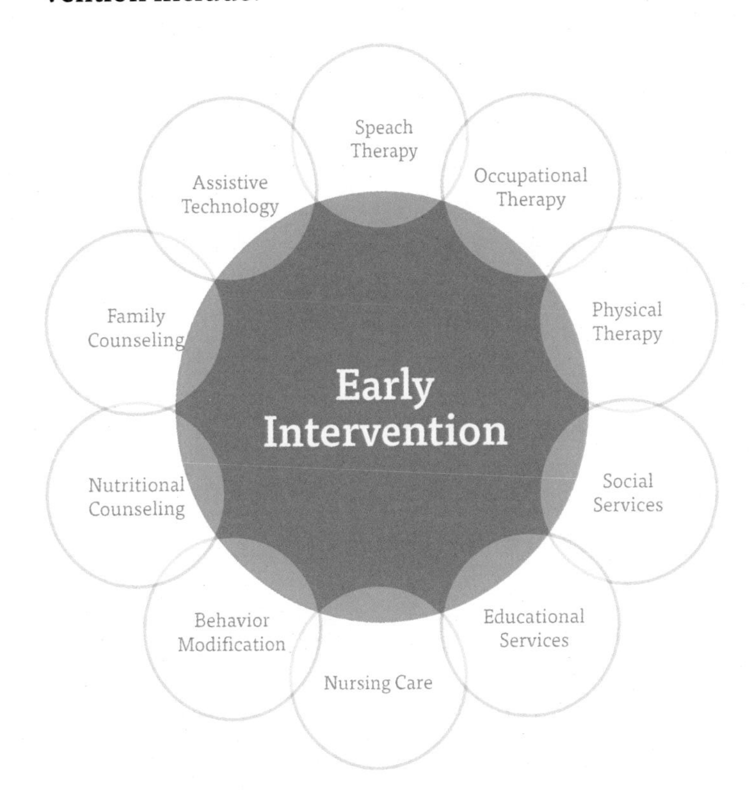

What Happens After Your Child Qualifies for EI?
Once your child has had an evaluation and it has been determined that they qualify for your state's EI services, you and your team of professionals will develop an Individualized Family Service Plan (IFSP). This plan outlines the services your child and family will receive through Early Intervention.

Daycare and Preschool

Many parents look for childcare and preschool programs for a variety of reasons. Unfortunately, when you have a child with special needs, you often have fewer choices. However, with increased awareness and guidance from the federal government about including children with special needs into preschool programs, positive change is on the horizon.

Under The Individuals with Disabilities and Education Act (IDEA) children have access to free public special education services outside of the home (drop-off programs) beginning at age three (may be earlier in some states). Before this time, there can be some hurdles to overcome when trying to find the right people and place to care for your child. Sometimes the search requires more work depending on how familiar people and places are with inclusion and ADA guidelines. If you get discouraged contact your local Department of Social Services and ask for assistance. The key is finding a facility with the desire and willingness to work with your child and family even if they do not yet know how. Once you have accomplished this, you may call upon a representative from a local or national organization (such as KIT–Kids Included Together) to help get the childcare team and family working together.

Many states offer additional funds to facilities caring for a child who has special needs. Check with your state's Department of Human Services about special needs child care subsidies.

Spread the word that you are looking for help. Talk to other parents (particularly those people who have children with special needs), social workers, doctors, or whomever you know that is a good source of information related to caring for your

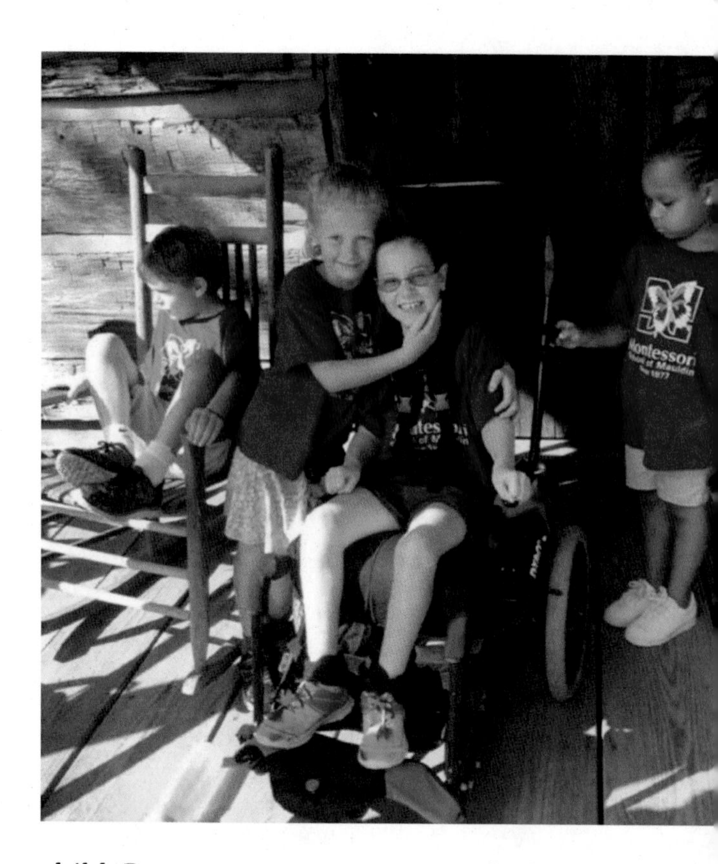

child. Parent-to-parent groups and other advocacy organizations may have a list of centers and people they have already worked with to establish inclusive programs.

You may have to have some flexibility with your expectations about the kind of daycare or preschool program you send your child to perhaps in regards to distance from your home, type of educational program, religious affiliation etc. However, do not let that flexibility include a potential compromise of your child's safety. Begin by making a list of what you are looking for in a facility. Determine what additional equipment, assistance or care your child may need to ensure their safety, comfort and sociability. Be honest about your child's needs and capabilities. Ultimately, you want to give the staff the opportunity to equip and educate themselves about how to best care for and teach/nurture your child. Always visit the facilities that interest you and eventually bring your child there before making a decision.

Questions to Ask

The following questions may be helpful to ask preschool and daycare program directors:

1. Has your facility ever cared for or had children with special needs?
2. If so, have any of these children ever had a physical disability?
3. Do you know or understand what cerebral palsy is?
4. Is your staff willing or open to learning about how to best care for my child?
5. Is your facility accessible to wheelchair users? Are there any areas that are not accessible?
6. How do you typically communicate with parents about their children and how often?
7. How closely would you be willing to communicate with me about concerns or issues that may arise with my child?
8. Would you allow my child's therapist/s to visit the facility and offer guidance about how to best support my child here?
9. Would you allow my child's therapists to come into the facility and conduct therapy with my child? **This is very convenient if the facility does not offer on-site therapy. It will save you time in the car traveling from one therapy appointment to the next.
10. Are you nervous about having my child attend here? If so, can we talk about your concerns?

**Many people are uneducated about CP, and may not understand that individual needs vary. If a facility is hesitant or nervous about including your child, remember that they may not have accurate information about CP, or are not used to accommodating children with special needs. Their initial response may be made up of fear or misunderstanding so it is important to educate administrators about your child's particular needs through open and honest conversation.

Blog Posts and Resources by Parents

- "5 signs of a good school for kids with special needs" by Ellen Seidman who blogs at *Love That Max*.
- Julie who blogs at *Have Wheelchair Will Travel*, offers her reflections on finding the right preschool for her son--now 18 years old in, "How Could You Not Want My Child?".

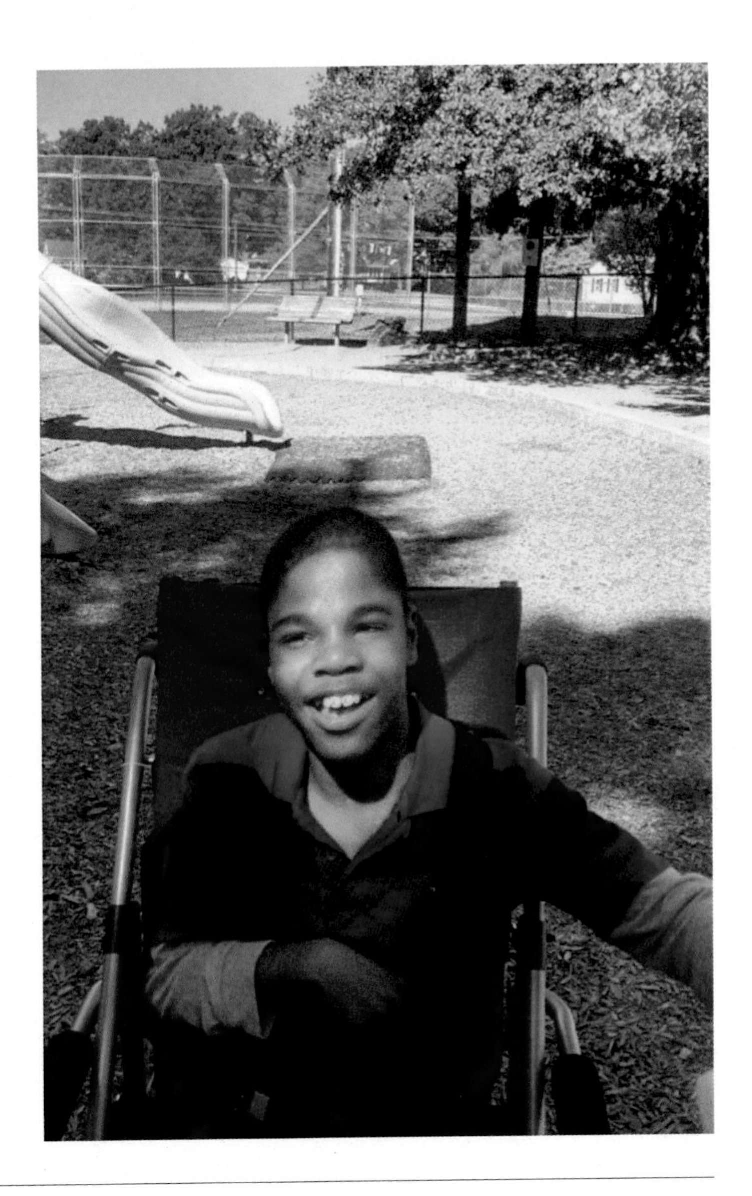

SECTION 8

Thinking Through Treatments

Treating CP is Not One Size Fits All

SINCE THE SYMPTOMS AND SEVERITY OF CP VARY GREATLY, TREATMENTS RECOMMENDED FOR SOME PEOPLE WITH CP MAY NOT BE RECOMMENDED FOR OTHERS AND EACH PERSON MAY RESPOND DIFFERENTLY. It is also important to consider conditions beyond problems with movement, balance, and coordination because these conditions may impact how treatments are evaluated for your child. These include problems with vision, learning, behavior, hearing, epilepsy, sensory integration, early or late onset of puberty, and others.

Often parents are anxious for new and better treatments and may be especially prone to try treatments based on unsubstantiated or scientifically unsound claims of therapeutic benefit. **It is important to take your time with treatment decisions.** As you hear about treatments for cerebral palsy make sure you are considering the specific symptoms you wish to address for your child and discuss how to best address them with your professional team.

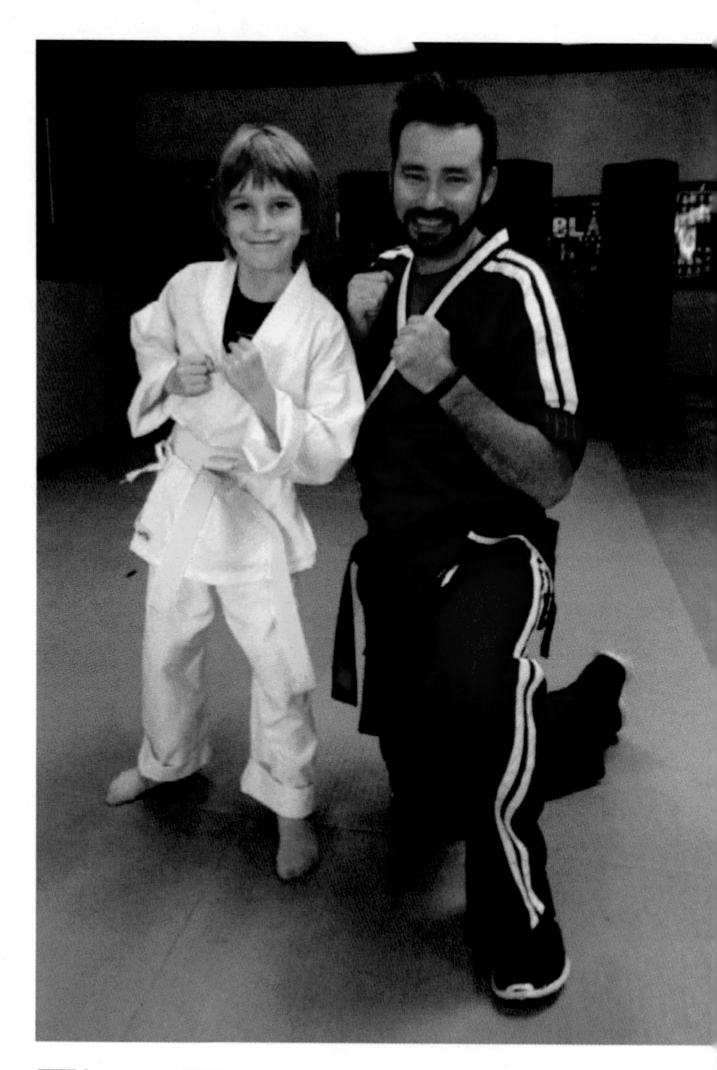

The Treatment Decision Checklist

This list is designed to help get you started with your treatment decision-making process. Ultimately, families have to determine their comfort level in pursuing any treatment whether it is well-established and widely researched, or if it is a new, experimental, or an "off-label" treatment. These are very personal decisions but, hopefully, the following considerations will empower and encourage you to have more in-depth discussions with your family and professional care team.

1. **Has the treatment being suggested been studied in people with CP?** The best evidence is based on studies of people of the same age range and diagnosis, and GMFCS level, and derived from sound, scientific research that is published in peer-reviewed journals.

2. **Has the treatment been evaluated on people or just animals?** A treatment that works on animals may or may not work on humans.

3. **Is the evidence based on a treatment that is clearly defined?** What does the treatment claim to do, and will this lead to accomplishing the goals you and/or your child have in mind? What evidence is there to show that the treatment makes a difference for the specific goals the family is trying to accomplish?

4. **Has the treatment been tried on a reasonable number of people?** Things that work on one, two or a handful of people could have happened by chance or for unrecognized reasons that are not going to apply to other people.

5. **In the evidence cited, has the treatment group of CP patients been compared to a similar group of CP patients who did not get the treatment?** How recent is the evidence?

6. **Could the evidence about a treatment really just be a "placebo effect?"**—that is when people say they are better just because they expect to be better and not because of any real effect of the treatment. The placebo effect is not necessarily a bad thing, and it's quite powerful. However, it is important to consider if positive outcomes from a treatment are stronger than a placebo effect.

7. **What costs are associated with the treatment and is it affordable?** Give this serious consideration, as new treatments, especially those sold on the internet may be very expensive and have hidden costs. Are there other, cheaper or more conventional treatment options that are as effective? Insurance companies are understandably wary of paying for treatments whose benefits are not scientifically substantiated.

8. **What is the cost in terms of time?** Consider the amount of time required to participate in the treatment and decide whether your time with your child may be better spent in other ways (play, travel, reading with them, and so on). Some programs may be impractical when one considers the impact on the whole family.

9. **What are the goals for a specific person with CP?** Are the goals realistic? How will you evaluate these goals? Will you compare the information before and after the treatment? And what is the time frame that you will use to evaluate these goals to determine if the treatment is helpful and worth your time and money?

Keep in mind that no known reputable treatment is appropriate and works on 100 percent of people. Be wary of any treatment that claims it is effective for all people with CP. Approach new treatments cautiously and with hopeful skepticism. If a treatment has a negative impact on the person's quality of life, you should seriously consider why you wish to continue.

SECTION 9

Treatments/ Interventions Glossary

AN IMPORTANT NOTE ABOUT THIS SECTION: This glossary includes *some* examples of commonly considered interventions for the primary movement disorder symptoms of CP—spasticity, dyskinesia and ataxia. Multiple treatments and therapies may be combined to address your child's symptoms and to support their development. Since there are many ways CP may affect the body, and a diversity of potential secondary conditions, it is not possible to introduce all potential treatments that may be relevant to your child in the CP Tool Kit. The definitions and information presented here are intended to provide a starting point for learning about potential CP treatments.

You are likely to hear different opinions and acceptance of these and other potential treatments and procedures. It is important to be a thoughtful consumer and ask your medical and professional team about their thinking and approach to the treatments they present and what evidence has led them to those opinions. Discuss the quality of existing evidence, potential risks and your doctor's confidence in a particular treatment being able to meet your child's and family's specific goals.

PT, OT, and Speech

(used for all types of CP)

Early in this journey, your child will be referred for therapy services in one more of the following modalities: Physical Therapy, Occupational Therapy and/or Speech Therapy. These three therapies are the most commonly prescribed, are covered by insurance (or through Early Intervention benefits) and are provided in your home, school or in an outpatient setting. These are broad categories under which there are many tools and specific approaches that therapists trained in these fields may use to help your child.

The purpose of therapy for your child is different than if we as adults need PT, OT or Speech. Adults go to therapy for "rehabilitation," to help us regain skills or movements that we had prior to an accident or injury. Children with CP go to therapy so they can learn new skills that they have not yet mastered and to learn adaptive skills to optimize their functional abilities. This is called "habilitation."

Your child may be prescribed therapy for a certain frequency (i.e number of times per week) and duration, but what your child works on in therapy is expected to be reinforced and practiced in the home, at school and in the community. It is very important that you be an active partner with your child and their therapist so that you can help them achieve the skills that they are working on. However, it is possible to overdo it. See "Creating a Balanced Therapy Program."

Physical Therapy (PT)

Physical therapy addresses the child's general strength, gross motor skills and mobility. Gross motor skills involve the large muscles of the body. Initial evaluations for physical therapy include

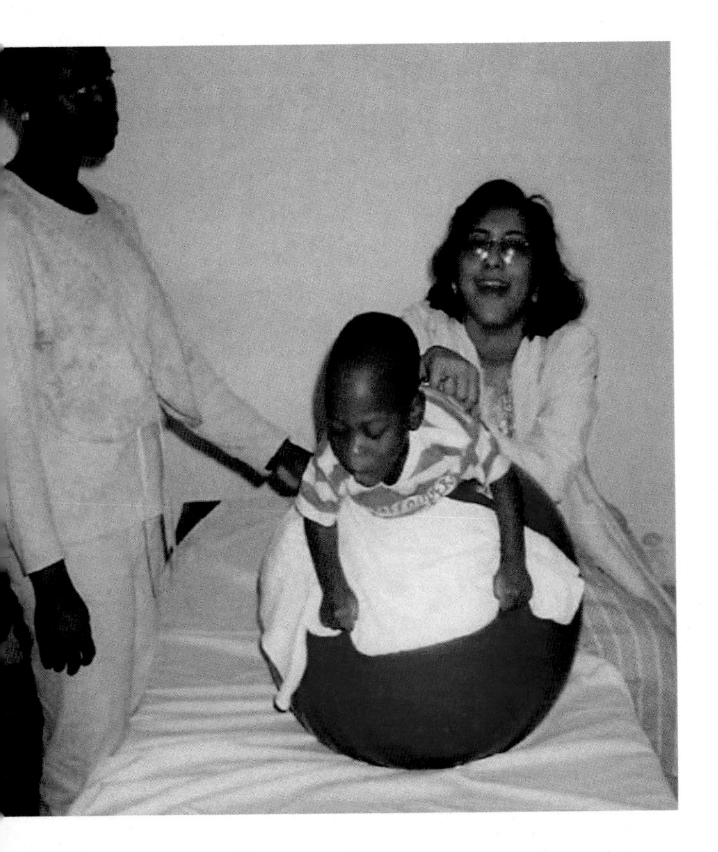

looking at the child's posture, sensory processing, muscle tone, coordination, developmental skills and adaptive equipment.

For cerebral palsy, there are primary impairments, such as spasticity, quality of movement and postural stability. There are also secondary impairments which are the result of how the primary impairments affect the body and they include things like reduced strength, range of motion limitations and problems with endurance. **PTs can help address the secondary impairments of CP. The therapist will help you target body structures and function in order to increase your child's activity and participation.** There are a few different models for providing PT.

Direct physical therapy goals and activities are individually established based on the evaluation and input from the family. They may include learning to sit, crawl, walk, climb steps, or throw or catch a ball. Activities include exercises for strengthening, range of motion and balance. Simple ball games, tricycle riding and outdoor play are used to improve coordination and endurance. Physical therapists often work with the family and local medical equipment vendors to identify, order, and maintain adaptive equipment to assist the child's sitting stability, posture, and/or mobility. Typical equipment includes orthotics, activity chairs, car seats, walkers, special strollers and wheelchairs. Physical therapists also work with the child's physicians when the child has skin problems—from lack of movement, contractures, or other orthopedic problems.

It's helpful for parents to become familiar with the GMFCS scale which is mentioned in the "Screenings and Assessments" section. This scale was developed as an objective way to assess gross motor function in children with CP and to set goals. It's intended to replace the very subjective terms of "mild", "moderate" and "severe."

Does your child have dyskinesia? spasticity? low muscle tone? A little of each?

The following are some commonly used approaches and support roles of physical therapists treating people with CP. Each therapist will differ slightly in their education, training and preferences for how they wish to approach treating the individual.

1. Resistance/Strength training
2. Functional balance training
3. Coordination exercises
4. Treadmill/Gait training
5. Robotics—robotic assisted movement—i.e. the Lokomat
6. Endurance training
7. Sports skills training
8. Stretching
9. Support with adaptive and assistive equipment selection and fitting
10. Aquatic Exercise Therapy

Occupational Therapy (OT)

Occupational Therapy (OT) refers to all of the "jobs" that make up daily life. An OT evaluates a child's ability to perform self-care, play and work/-school skills. These are referred to as ADL's-activities of daily living. Through a comprehensive evaluation, the OT can identify issues that interfere with a child's completion of these many skills/tasks. These may include problems with strength, abnormal muscle tone, eye-hand coordination, visual perceptual skills, and sensory processing skills. The goal of OT is for the child to participate as actively and independently as possible in all areas of ADL. Therapy is child-directed and based on activities that are meaningful and purposeful to that specific child and the child's family.

OTs also assess whether adaptive equipment and assistive technology may increase a child's independence. Examples include specialized feeding utensils, switches to access computers and electronics, adaptive scissors and writing utensils, splints, and adaptations to clothing such as zipper pulls and button hooks. Pediatric OTs may also provide constraint therapy, sensory integrative (SI) therapy, vision related therapies and feeding related therapy.

Speech-Language Therapy

See also Assistive technology

Speech pathologists can foster communication between parents/caregivers and children even when there is little verbal speech. This may include: pre-language skills (vocalizations), manual sign language, gestures, picture communication boards, and/or voice output communication devices. These strategies for communicating can reduce your child's frustration, and increase their opportunities for self-expression.

Strategies:

LANGUAGE INTERVENTION ACTIVITIES — The SLP will interact with a child by playing and talking, using pictures, books, objects, or ongoing events to stimulate language development. The therapist may also model correct pronunciation and use repetition exercises to build speech and language skills.

ARTICULATION THERAPY — Articulation, or sound production, exercises involve having the therapist model correct sounds and syllables for a child, often during play activities. The level of play is age-appropriate and related to the child's specific needs. The SLP will physically show the child how to make certain sounds, such as the "r" sound, and may demonstrate (in front of a mirror) how to move the tongue to produce specific sounds.

ORAL-MOTOR/FEEDING AND SWALLOWING THERAPY — The SLP will use a variety of oral exercises — including facial massage and various tongue, lip, and jaw exercises to strengthen the muscles of the mouth. The SLP also may work with different food textures and temperatures to increase a child's oral awareness during eating and swallowing.

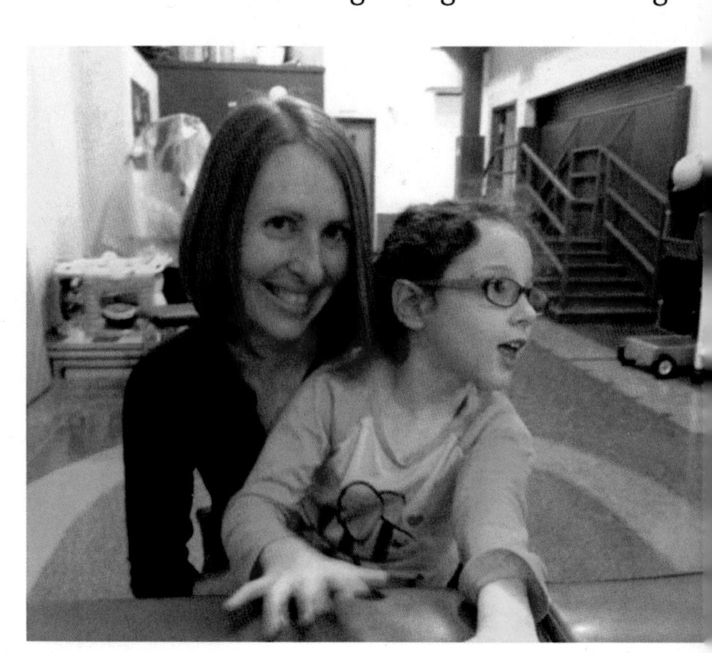

AUGMENTATIVE/ALTERNATIVE COMMUNICATION (AAC) — AAC is used to describe any form other than talking to communicate. Communication boards, charts and/or sign language are often beginning options to support communication for young children. As your child grows, specialized communication programs can be used on a computer, an i-Pad, or other tablet devices. These devices allow for flexibility in access, meaning they have multiple ways for your child to use them beyond typing. AAC systems allow for both speech and written communication.

Here is an extraordinary TED talk about the importance of fostering communication from an adult with CP who had lots to say but no way to say it until he was 6 years old!

Treatments by Movement Disorder Type

The Treatment Glossary continues here with some commonly considered interventions for the **movement disorders of CP**. There may be several approaches to addressing the same problem, and each may have varying amounts of evidence for effectiveness, safety, and how well they have been proven to meet specific treatment goals.

Some families may pursue treatments to manage pain or to prevent contractures. Others may be more focused on making caregiving routines (i.e diapering, toileting, dressing, and bathing) easier or improving functional outcomes like walking or sitting. In some cases, especially medications, there may evidence for use in other populations, but not in people with CP, and maybe not in children. It is important to speak with your medical team about these and other issues including side effects, your treatment goals, required follow-up care, and whether your child is an appropriate candidate for a particular treatment or procedure. At times it may be helpful to get multiple professional opinions and speak with other families who have had the procedures you are considering. You need to ensure you have clarity and comfort in moving forward with any treatment or procedure.

Spasticity treatment options

Spasticity in CP is typically addressed by using different ways to disrupt or counterbalance the messages sent from the brain to the muscles that are causing spasticity. This can be done through oral medications, implantable medications, and through a variety of surgical procedures on the spinal nerves, muscles and tendons. More than one approach may be used together to manage symptoms associated with spasticity.

What is botulinum toxin?

Botulinum toxin, is a chemical produced by the bacteria clostridium botulinum. In CP, it may be injected into specific muscles to temporarily relax stiff or spastic muscles by blocking the connection between a nerve and the muscle. It is thought that decreasing muscle stiffness may allow for better stretching of shortened muscles. It also may provide relief from pain from muscle tightness.

Over the last 25 years, botulinum toxin has been commonly used to treat neuromuscular conditions including spasticity. However, it was only in 2016, the US Food and Drug Administration (FDA) gave its first approval for a brand of botulinum toxin A called Dysport, to be used in children with CP. Dysport has been approved for the use in the treatment of lower limb muscle stiffness in CP, and specifically a pediatric population of 2 years and older.

It is very important to discuss the specific indications for use of botulinum toxin and its potential risks with your medical team. There are several formulations and strains (usually A or B used in CP) of botulinum toxin that are commonly used *"off-label" by physicians. In addition, the 2016 approval for Dysport (botulinum toxin A) was based on a study that included a specific population within CP and with specific indications for use.

In 2009 the FDA issued a Boxed Warning for botulinum toxin (available for review on the FDA website). Discuss this warning, other potential side effects, risks and appropriate candidacy with your medical team.

What are ethanol/phenol nerve blocks?

Nerve blocking using ethanol or phenol is used as a way of reducing spasticity (muscle tightness) by blocking the overactive nerve signal from the brain to a group of muscles that the nerve connects to. This is done by dissolving the myelin sheath (fatty coating) wrapped around the nerve. This approach requires more precision than the use of botulinum toxin since specific nerves are being targeted rather than larger muscles. The effects of the injection typically wear off once the nerve regenerates which can vary widely from one person to another.

Discuss potential side effects, risks and appropriate candidacy with your medical team.

What is a baclofen pump?

The baclofen pump is a refillable, programmable pump that contains the medication baclofen. Baclofen is used to reduce excessive muscle tone for spasticity and symptoms of dystonia. The baclofen pump is typically implanted under the skin or muscles toward the front of the abdominal wall. It delivers the baclofen medication via an implanted catheter that is inserted into the spine. This is called intrathecal baclofen. By administering the medication into the spinal canal the medication does not circulate throughout the body first and smaller doses of the medication are needed. This potentially reduces some of the side effects, or the intensity of side effects, commonly associated with taking oral baclofen.

A screening test using oral baclofen or a one time intrathecal dose is usually performed prior to the placement of the pump. This will help determine if the individual will respond to intrathecal baclofen. Once implanted, follow-up medical care is needed approximately every three to six months to refill medication in the pump. After five to seven years, at the end of the pumps battery life, the pump is replaced.

Discuss potential side effects, risks and appropriate candidacy with your medical team.

What is selective dorsal rhizotomy (SDR)?

SDR is a surgical procedure intended to reduce muscle spasticity in patients with CP. An incision is made along the center of the lower back. Once the spinal nerves are visible the surgical team identifies the sensory rootlets causing spasticity (they test the nerves to evaluate their level of activity) and they sever the abnormal rootlets. Intensive post surgical physical therapy is required and individuals must be carefully evaluated for their candidacy. Typically people with CP who have multiple movement disorders are not considered to be suitable candidates.

Discuss potential side effects, risks and appropriate candidacy with your medical team.

*"Off-label" refers to the use of a medication outside the specifications outlined in the FDA's approved medication packaging label or insert. "Off-label" prescribing is legal and common in medicine since the cost associated with each FDA approval for a drug is many millions of dollars. Ideally, we would have studies for how a specific population with a specific indication responds to every drug, but the cost and rigor of the process make it an insurmountable expectation. Regardless, it's important to understand this concept and determine your comfort level when selecting treatments. Always discuss potential risks/benefits with your medical team.

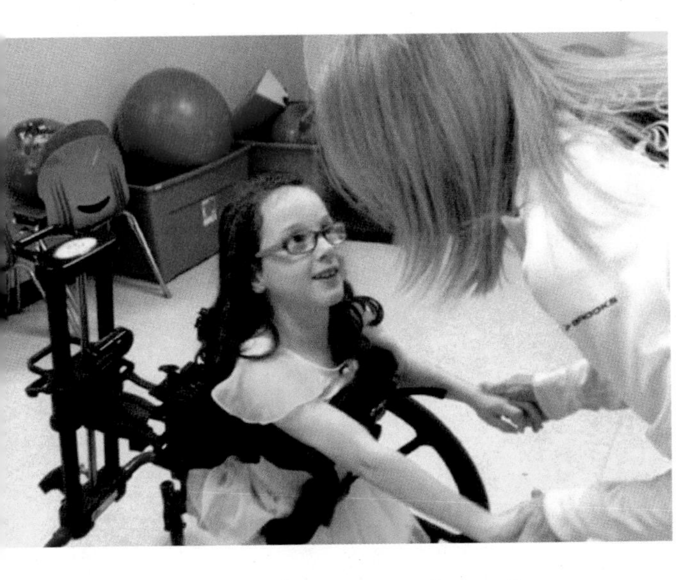

What are lengthening procedures?

Lengthening procedures of the muscles or tendons are surgical procedures that may be considered to reduce spasticity, address contractures, improve range of motion and in some cases reduce pain. There are many ways to lengthen a muscle, depending on the type and location of the muscle, and the extent to which it must be lengthened. The muscles may be detached from their connection to the bone, the tendons or tissue of the tendons may be divided or cut, or the myofascia (muscle fascia) maybe be divided. The myofascia is a sheet of tendon-like material, mainly serving to connect a muscle with the parts it moves.

Common muscles/tendons that are lengthened include the muscles in the back of the calf including the Achilles tendon (heel cord), the hamstring muscles/tendons behind the knee, and the adductor muscles in the groin. Lengthening of muscles and tendons are intended to improve the range of motion, but will also weaken the muscle considerably, if the amount of lengthening is excessive.

Discuss potential side effects, risks and appropriate candidacy with your medical team.

What are tendon transfer procedures?

In CP, not all muscles around a joint are equally affected by increased tone. It is not uncommon to find some muscles are affected by spasticity, while their counterparts (antagonist muscle) on the other side of the joint are weak. Consequently, joint deformity can occur due to the over-activity of one group of muscles overpowering another group. Under these circumstances, the deformity can be addressed by transferring part or all of tendon of the overactive or spastic muscle and redirecting it and reattaching it to the other side of the joint to balance the forces around that joint.

Discuss potential side effects, risks and appropriate candidacy with your medical team.

Medications (Oral)

Some medications you may hear about to treat spasticity include **oral baclofen, diazepam (Valium), tizanidine (Zanaflex)** and **dantrolene (Dantrium)**. **Gabapentin (Neurontin)** is also sometimes used to treat pain associated with spasticity. In the case of oral baclofen, patients who have had success but end up with too many side effects, may be presented with information about the baclofen pump (mentioned above) which may offer the benefits of the higher doses of the medication with potentially fewer side effects. At the same time the baclofen pump has its own potential side effects and contraindications which differ from the oral medication.

Discuss potential side effects, risks, "off-label" use and appropriate candidacy with your medical team.

Dyskinesia treatment options: DYSTONIA, CHOREA and ATHETOSIS

Dystonia treatment options:

A baclofen pump (as discussed in the spasticity treatment section) may be considered by providers for the treatment of secondary dystonia—dystonia due to cerebral palsy—particularly after medications have been tried. It is not FDA approved yet for this indication (but has been for spasticity).

Discuss potential side effects, risks, "off-label" use and appropriate candidacy with your medical team.

What is deep brain stimulation (DBS)?

DBS delivers electrical impulses, through electrodes implanted within specific areas of the brain. It has been used to treat neurological conditions such as essential tremor, Parkinson's and certain forms of dystonia, particularly genetic forms. Currently deep brain stimulation is being explored as a potential treatment for dyskinetic forms of cerebral palsy but more research is needed, particularly for use in children. Since there are very limited treatment options available for dystonia due to CP, we chose to highlight DBS here for you to discuss developments in research with your medical team.

Discuss potential side effects, risks and appropriate candidacy with your medical team.

Medications (Oral)

Some medications that you may hear about as a potential treatment of dystonia in CP include **trihexyphenidyl (Artane)**, **L-dopa** or **carbidopa-levodopa (Sinemet)**, **clonazepam (Klonopin)**. Research in other populations have shown **tetrabenazine (Xenazine)** and **zolpidem (Ambien)** to be effective in treating some forms of dystonia.

Stay connected with us to learn how you can help advocate to advance research and treatments for CP. Discuss potential side effects, risks, "off-label" use and appropriate candidacy with your medical team.

Chorea treatment options

Medications (Oral)

Tetrabenazine (Xenazine) is FDA approved to treat Chorea associated with Huntington's disease but has not been specifically studied in people who have chorea due to cerebral palsy. Stay connected with us to learn how you can help advocate to advance research and treatments for CP.

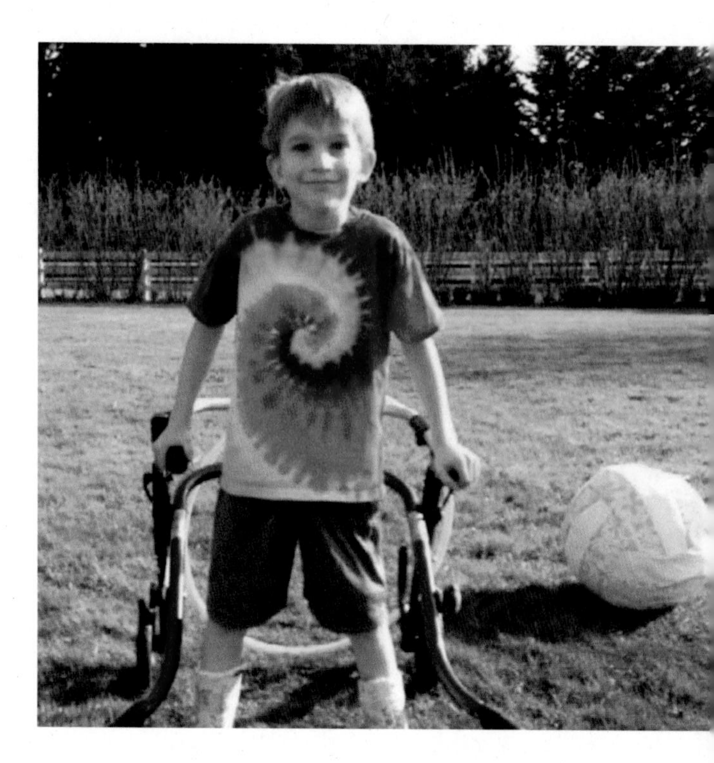

Discuss potential side effects, risks, "off-label" use and appropriate candidacy with your medical team.

Athetosis treatment options

No effective and widely utilized treatments known at this time—Stay connected with us to learn how you can help advocate to advance research and treatments for CP.

Ataxia treatment options

No effective and widely utilized treatments known at this time—Stay connected with us to learn how you can help advocate to advance research and treatments for CP.

Mixed CP treatment options

Treatment for mixed forms of CP is often approached by addressing the symptoms of the individual movement disorders. As an example, an individual may take medications to address he movement disorder of dystonia but also may consider others interventions such as botulinum toxin or a soft tissue lengthening to address issues related to spasticity. Treating mixed CP is a balance that can often be difficult to achieve and must be revisited often as your child grows and changes. Sometimes, for example, an effort to reduce spasticity may reveal underlying muscle weakness or more dystonia, which in-turn needs to be addressed by your child's treatment team either through therapy, medication adjustments, or equipment adjustments.

General Orthopedic Procedures for CP

As mentioned previously, when someone has CP the brain sends confusing signals to the muscles. This then affects the individual's ability to control and move small and large muscles throughout the body. As the child grows the muscles may not stretch and grow at the pace at which the bones are growing. This can place abnormal stress on the bones and skeleton in a variety of ways potentially affecting alignment, posture, and the shape of the bones. Some of these orthopedic topics were discussed in the "Early Screenings and Assessments" portion of the Tool Kit. Below are a couple examples of orthopedic procedures that may be used to address some of the secondary musculoskeletal conditions commonly seen in people who have CP. There are many others not mentioned here that may be pertinent to addressing your child's symptoms. Consult with your medical team for further information.

Addressing contractures

Lengthening procedures of the muscles or tendons are surgical procedures that can be used to correct contractures—reduced range of movement of the joints caused by shortened muscles. Contractures can be caused by increased muscle tone due to spasticity but can also occur in the presence of normal muscle tone or even low muscle tone (due to less mobility and therefore less stretching of the muscle). At the point when a contracture becomes "fixed" surgery may be suggested since it is less likely to respond to muscle tone management strategies such as medications or the use of botox.

Discuss potential side effects, risks and appropriate candidacy with your medical team.

Bony deformities in CP—What is an osteotomy?

Osteotomy is the term for surgical correction of a bony deformity. In CP osteotomies are commonly performed on the hips, knees, and/or ankles. In growing children the shape of the bones (particularly in the legs) changes naturally over time. This happens in response to gravitational forces acting upon the bones as the child moves through motor milestones such as sitting, crawling and walking. In children who have CP, these milestones are delayed or may not be achieved, and consequently the child's bones may resemble more of their original shape from birth. This may lead to joints (such as the hip) becoming unstable and can affect the quality and efficiency of walking.

For instance, the infant thigh bone (femur) has an internal twist (anteversion), which typically unwinds by walking age. The persistence of this twist and other aspects of the shape of the thigh bone near the hip make it more prone to hip displacement and dislocation, a common problem in CP. In cases such as these there comes a point where an osteotomy may be presented to address this problem by reconstructing the hips.

Sometimes muscle/tendon lengthening procedures, tendon transfers and osteotomies, are performed under the same anesthetic to address all the contractures and bone deformities at once. This is called **multilevel surgery**.

Not all children with CP are candidates for orthopaedic surgery, and the type and timing of surgery can depend on many factors. In general, surgery is avoided if possible in the youngest children, to avoid the possibility of recurrent deformities that might need additional surgery in the future.

"The whole is greater than the sum of its parts." *Aristotle*

Although CP has been recognized and featured in the medical literature for more than a century, there are many aspects about these movement disorders that are not yet well understood. Because of this lack of understanding, many of the above treatments that address the individual symptoms of the movement disorders may only incrementally help your child achieve their functional goals. For example, lessening spasticity and relaxing tight muscles that may be interfering with movement does not always lead to an improved gait or easier sitting. There could be many possible reasons for this related to the complexity of brain development and how movement is created that we are still learning about.

Complementary or Alternative Medicines (CAMs)

Many families who have children with CP explore complementary or alternative medicines (CAMs). CAMs cover a wide range of topics and ideas. They can be therapies or movement programs such as hydrotherapy, yoga, Feldenkrais or therapeutic riding. These kinds of programs are CAMS that may complement or support a traditional therapy or treatment program by providing opportunities for moving in ways that may be fun or relaxing, but perhaps have not been proven to specifically address the symptoms of CP. There are also experimental treatments like stem cells where there are still many questions about safety and/or proof of benefit. Other treatments, such as hyperbaric oxygen therapy (HBOT) have not been embraced by many mainstream physicians because there is a large body of research which has shown that HBOT is no more effective than placebo in addressing the symptoms of CP. For these reasons it is important to identify what you mean when using the term "CAMs" and the specific goals you wish to accomplish in pursuing CAMs for treatment.

For instance are you searching for pain relief, better range of motion, improved balance, an activity that provides relaxation? Or are you looking for more drastic changes in mobility? Many CAMs like yoga have anecdotal evidence to support their use in CP and offer great opportunities for movement and exercise. In something like acupuncture there is a large body of research and a 5000-year history to support its use for general pain relief. However, these treatments may not have been extensively researched in people with CP and formally proven to help with things like spasticity or fine motor control.

What makes CAMs appealing to parents?

- Excitement about new ideas
- Belief in "natural" things
- Hearing testimonials/stories about an alternative treatment or program (i.e My friend's son did this or used this and this great result occurred.)
- Frustration with slow pace of child's developmental changes, and with emerging research breakthroughs

On the internet, there are many anecdotal reports and promotional claims about various treatments for CP. However, many of these treatments, do not stand up to rigorous scientific investigation or have not been tested yet. It is important to be objective. Consider the potential risks along with the potential benefits so that you will not be spending lots of time, money, and false hope unnecessarily. In addition, some treatments may harm the child. **Unknown risks do not mean that risks do not exist.** For example, "natural things" such as dietary supplements and herbal products may interact with other products or medications a child with CP may be taking. They also may have unwanted side effects on their own. Seek information and insight from professionals and people not associated with selling the product or therapy you are interested in pursuing.

Discussing CAMs can lead to heated discussions between professionals and parents. Approach these discussions objectively and with as much humility and honesty as possible so that everyone may learn from each other. Keep in mind that if you are doing more than one therapy or treatment at a time you may not know what changes to attribute to which treatment. For more information and ideas about how to think through treatment options refer back to the "Treatment Decision Checklist".

You may wish to watch this very informative CP-NET Webinar on Complementary and Alternative Therapies by Dr. Peter Rosenbaum, Co-founder of CanChild Centre in Canada. It discusses and critically analyzes the concept of complementary and alternative therapies.[24] **Please note this webinar is for educational purposes only. Consult with your medical team for specific guidance, potential risks and the most current research and information about treatments.

What about stem cells and CP?

Stem cells are the master cells of our bodies. They are how we grow new skin, hair and heal broken bones. All stem cells, regardless of their source in the body, have the potential to develop into many different cell types for use throughout the body, while also retaining their ability to produce more stem cells, a process called self-renewal.

Experiments over the last several years have shown that stem cells from one tissue may give rise to cell types of a completely different tissue. For example, a blood-forming adult stem cell (meaning non-embryonic) in the bone marrow normally gives rise to many types of blood cells. This means that it may be possible to use stem cells generally thought to be blood-forming stem cells for something like neurological repair. This is why stem cells are being explored as a potential treatment for CP. In theory these cells could potentially help repair and restore damaged tissue and connections in the brain.

Stem cell therapy remains an area of great debate within the research community. Additional research using adult stem cells is necessary to understand their full potential and safety as future therapies.

What research has been published on the use of stem cells as a treatment for CP?

It is still unknown whether stem cell treatment is a viable option for neurological repair. There are a few completed and ongoing stem cell trials for CP worldwide that are exploring the efficacy and safety of stem cells for people with cerebral palsy. The United States has a few current active stem cell studies. You may visit the following website www.clinicaltrials.gov and search for studies currently recruiting.

Additional educational resources on stem cells:

The ISSR (International Society for Stem Cell Research) website offers excellent information to help consumers understand more about stem cells and what is known currently about their potential applications in medicine.

Creating a Balanced Therapy Program

By Michele Shusterman

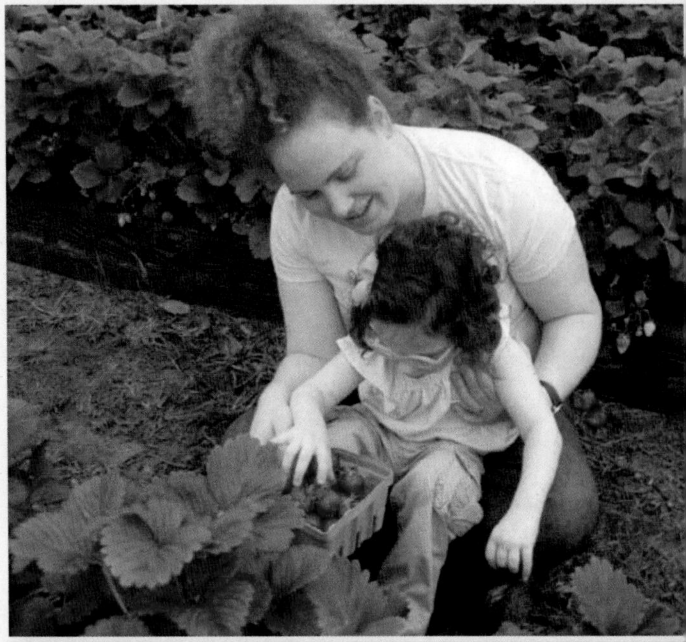

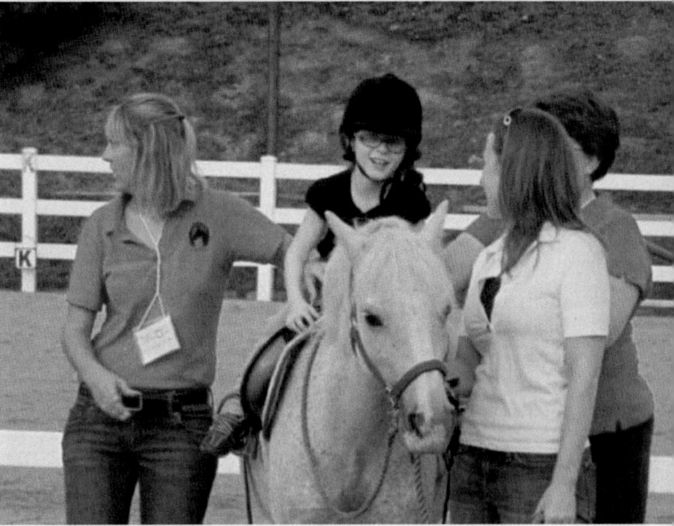

AS YOU BEGIN TO CONSIDER HOW TO HELP YOUR CHILD, many of you will feel overwhelmed when creating your child's therapy schedule. You may feel that there are not enough hours in the day or week to fit everything in for your child, your family and yourself. You are not alone in this feeling. This journey is not easy. We all face common fears and, perhaps, guilt around trying to do whatever we can to help our children. **Here are some things to think about as you create your child's therapy program.**

1 **Your child will have his or her own developmental timeline.** When you compare your child to other same aged peers, you may subliminally approach your child with disappointment and she may perceive this as something she is doing wrong. Focus on the positive points, what is working and the seemingly small, incremental steps that lead to putting larger developmental pieces together.

2 **Be honest and aware of what is driving your approach to creating your child's therapy program. Be on the lookout for guilt, fear, and hopelessness that leads you to push your child and other family members in unhealthy ways.** As one fellow parent said to me, "For me, trying to fix my child was the only way I could feel any ounce of control when the situation felt so completely out of control." Those words resonated with how I also felt in the first few years after my daughter was diagnosed with CP. I had to find some way to help my child and do whatever I could to make her path easier. This isn't necessarily a bad thing but it is important to be mindful of its influence on your decision-making.

3 **If you are trying a new therapy, make a list of what sacrifices you and your family will be making, including any emotional, physical, financial, or safety and unknown risks.** Remember that if the risks associated with a treatment are not known this does not mean the treatment will not potentially cause harm. Discuss these issues with people you

trust and your child's medical team. Set time commitment and financial limits and discuss expectations.

4 **Assess and honor your child's physical and cognitive energy limits each day.** These may change daily. You know your child best. Don't be afraid to speak up if you think what is best for your child is different from what the experts advise.

5 **Creating a balanced schedule will get easier as your child's developmental picture becomes clearer.** As your child gets older and your professional team has had more time to observe her, you will have a better understanding of what challenges you will be dealing with long-term.

6 **Carve out times during the day to simply be with your child, other family members, or spouse without thinking about CP, or assessing how your child is moving, speaking, walking, etc.**

7 **Focus on what your child does well and what she likes.** Integrate interests with opportunities for development. My daughter loves riding horses and to her it doesn't feel like work. The riding facility we go to recently referred to therapeutic riding as similar to sneaking broccoli into cookies and I couldn't agree more! Remember they are a child first, not a patient.

8 **There is no secret cure for CP. When there is a major breakthrough in symptoms or complete alleviation of them, it won't be a secret.**

I have definitely moved into a place of deeper acceptance of my daughter's obstacles, and I now spend much less of my time and energy thinking about how to make her symptoms of CP go away. By focusing on her accomplishments, I feel more optimistic and hopeful, rather than feeling hurried and guilty because I am not making enough happen for her. I look for smaller developmental changes, still hoping for the larger ones but not counting on them. I celebrate her triumphs alongside her. We spend much more time laughing and having fun. **It's taken time and work to reach this point and some days are better than others, but ultimately we are much happier and healthier as a family by focusing less on CP and more on living.**

Pace yourself—"Life is a marathon not a sprint."

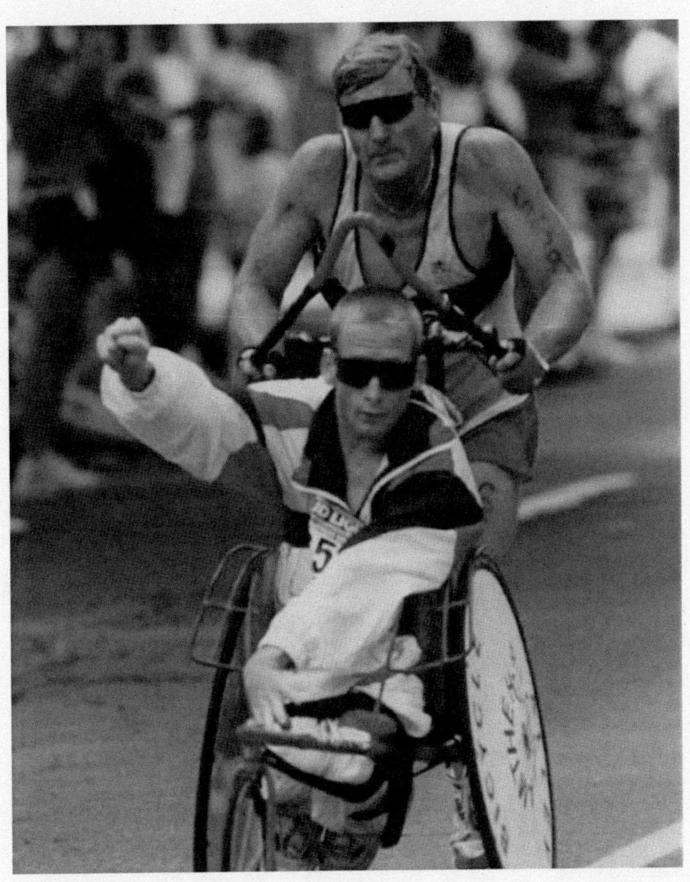

Permission for use of photo by Team Hoyt

Assistive Technology (AT)

AT services can open up many possibilities for people with CP to further engage in life by supporting communication, education, and better physical access to the world through the use of technology. Some examples of assistive technology include environmental control switches (to control the doors, lights, tv or toys), adapted keyboards and mice, visual aids and books on tape. Assistive technology provides the support that allows an individual to complete their intended action that their body may not be able to achieve or achieve easily. AT services can be provided by a variety of service professionals including speech therapists, vision professionals, PTs, OTs and teachers.

Equipment, Durable Medical Goods & Orthoses

There are many different kinds of equipment and supportive devices available for people with CP. It is important that the family and medical team determine the goals for the child and the needs of the caregiver when considering what equipment and supportive devices to explore. Mobility devices such as strollers, wheelchairs, power chairs and mobile standers, as well as personal care support, recreation equipment and orthoses (devices/braces) are among the things that can be helpful. The purpose of these devices is to encourage development and provide independence and/or support for engaging more comfortably and fully in daily activities.

Approach each equipment option as an extension of your child, helping them to access their environment, engage with their peers, and provide independence. Carefully selected equipment can open up important opportunities for your child and allow them to experience aspects of life and independent exploration they may otherwise miss. For example, children of walking age who are unable to walk should be given opportunities to be at peer level. If a child's peers are standing and walking around the classroom, and your child is on the floor they are likely having different learning experiences. By bringing them to the same height it opens up a sense of equality because they have more opportunities to learn and interact together.

Personal care is a part of life and there are options to offer your child as much independence as possible, especially as they grow. Hand rails or grab bars for the bathroom may be found at home improvement stores or also may possibly be ordered with insurance coverage under a policy's durable medical equipment allowance (check individual policies for more information). Be sure support bars are securely attached to the wall (via a studs that sits behind the wall), and per the manufacturer's instructions. You may wish to consult or hire a professional to perform the installation for you. There are also attachments for the toilet, bathing chairs and lifts to fit most bathrooms and personal needs.

Adaptive bicycles, jogging strollers and beach wheelchairs are **recreational equipment options** that are available. Although your insurance may not provide coverage for these options, there are organizations (such as some Easter Seals locations) with equipment lending closets that may be able to assist you.

Transporting your child as they grow can be a challenge. Car seats that swivel, portable ramps and transport vans are things to consider. Electronic lifts may also be added to a vehicle, or storage platforms can attach to the back of the vehicle to allow for wheelchair transport.

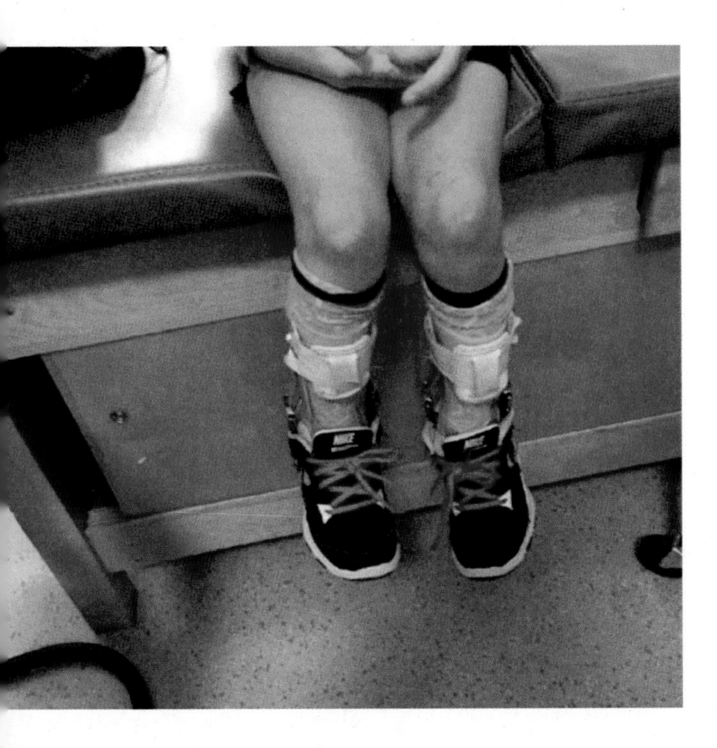

Orthoses fit onto the body and are used to encourage proper alignment and offer extra support to areas of the body with less tone (such as the trunk). Ankle/Foot Orthosis (AFO's) are one example of a commonly used orthosis in people with different types of CP. They are designed to aid foot and knee stability, ankle placement, walking efficiency, gait pattern and bone development. If your child needs an AFO or other orthotic, you will be referred to a podiatrist or orthotist who will create a cast of the foot/leg where the brace is needed. The cast will either be sent off to another company to make the AFO or the AFO will be made in the office.

Mobility equipment options such as adaptive strollers, walkers, wheelchairs and standers vary in size, so a consultation with a professional equipment vendor and your child's therapist is the most important part of ensuring a proper fit. There are a variety of mobility options available and your therapists or other medical professionals should assist in determining the best ones for your child.

Your insurance company may only cover select brands and/or accessory items depending on their cost. You should always consult with your insurance company and/or their Durable Medical

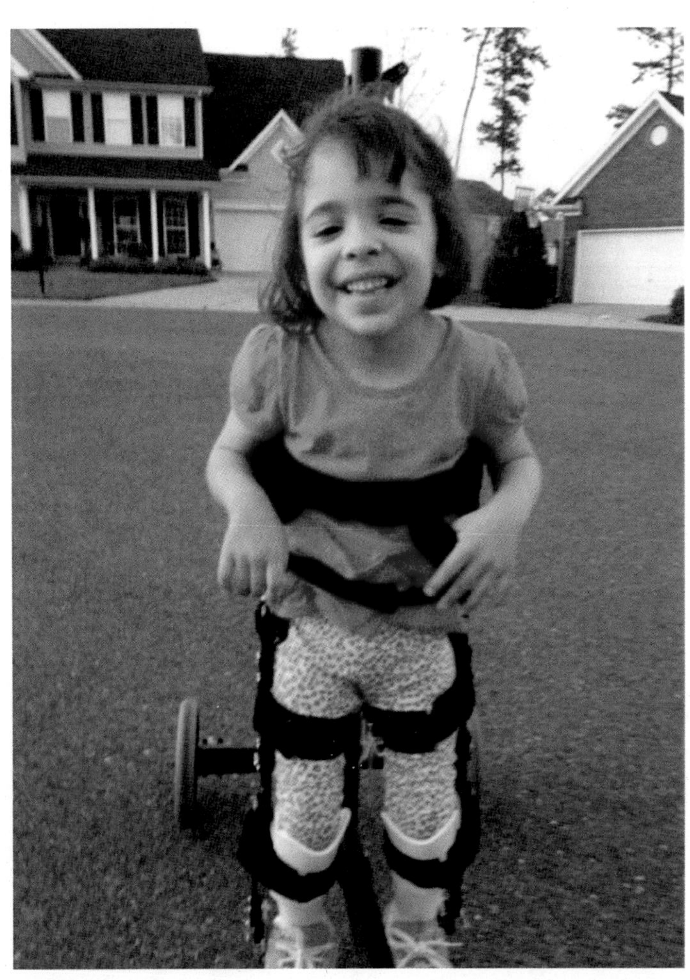

Equipment (DME) provider before making any purchases. Options such as transport ties—anchors used to secure wheelchairs while on a bus or in a vehicle—may be necessary items for your family, but some insurance companies do not cover them, leaving you responsible for the out-of-pocket expense.

It is important to thoroughly test equipment to make sure that it offers the benefits you are looking for and that your child is ready for and comfortable using the equipment to its full benefit. Many facilities, such as physical therapy offices, or local nonprofits have lending closets for you to try out different types of equipment. You or your therapist may also arrange for your equipment vendor to bring in demonstration models to test. **Take your time making decisions about equipment; many items are expensive investments that your child will be using for several years.**

SECTION 10

Insurance & Special Needs Planning

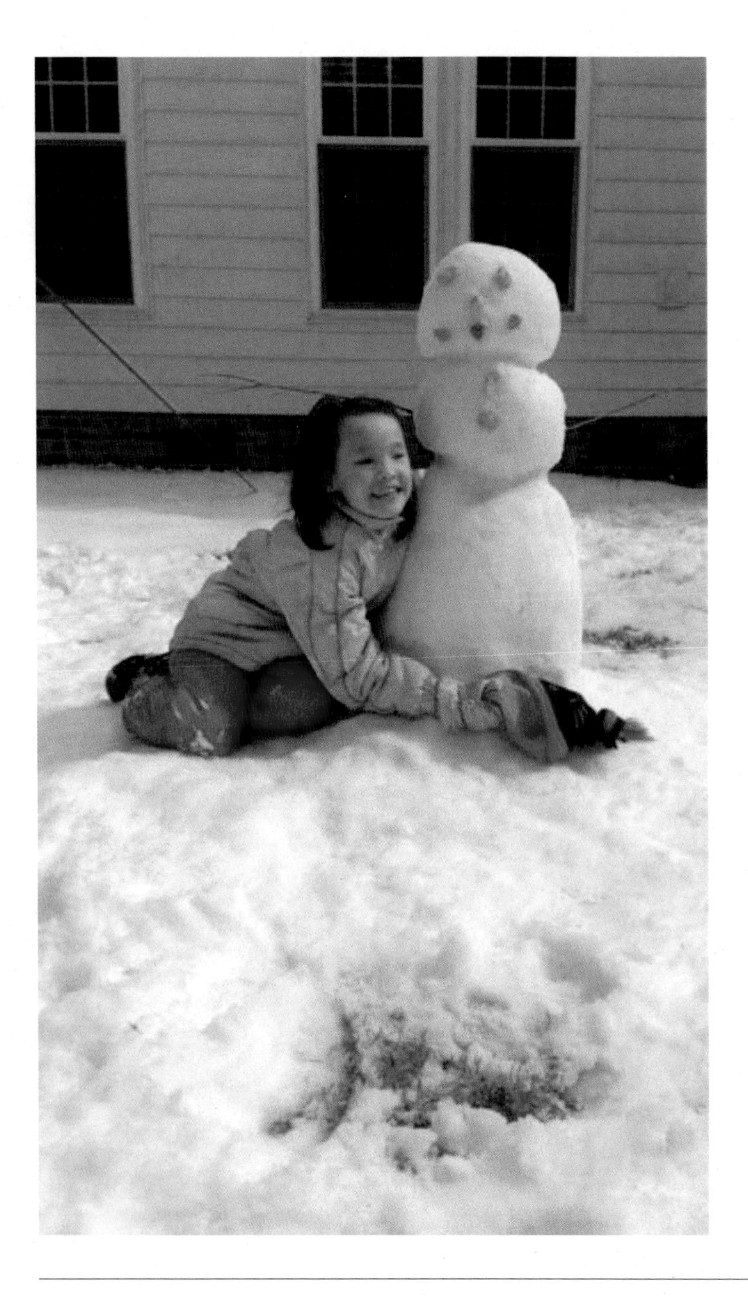

Health Insurance

FOR MANY FAMILIES raising a child with cerebral palsy, navigating the ins and outs of health insurance can be time consuming and confusing. It is likely that your child is covered as a dependent on your group health insurance, through an Affordable Care Act (ACA) plan https://www.healthcare.gov, independent plan or by Medicaid/CHIP. The ACA, gives parents more freedom to choose an insurance policy that best fits their needs because now there are no lifetime limits on the dollar value of insurance coverage, young adults are covered on their parent's plan up to age 26 and insurers are prohibited from cancelling coverage except in cases of fraud. The ACA also prohibits pre-existing condition exclusions. **Prior to the ACA, pre-existing condition exclusions were a significant barrier for individuals with CP.**

The intent of this section is to summarize what may be available to you in addition to your current health plan and to provide a few tips/tricks to help you navigate the complicated system of potential insurers. http://hdwg.org/catalyst/medicaid-tutorial

TEFRA — Tax Equity and Fiscal Responsibility Act of 1982

Allows states to extend Medicaid coverage to certain children with disabilities. TEFRA is a category of Medicaid that provides support and resources to families to care for their children in their homes (instead of a nursing home). Unlike traditional Medicaid, the TEFRA option does not consider parent resources when determining eligibility for program participation (the child's resources are considered). Currently 18 states and the District of Columbia offer TEFRA and several other states offer look-alike options. To qualify for TEFRA benefits, the child must be disabled according to the Supplemental Security Income (SSI) definition of disability and must meet the medical-necessity requirement for "institutional" care. (We don't care for this term but it is the technical definition.) Children who live in or receive extended care in nursing homes or long term care facilities are not eligible for TEFRA programs. http://www.hdwg.org/catalyst/cover-more-kids/tefra or http://www.hdwg.org/catalyst/TEFRA-FOA-worksheet

Medicaid/CHIP Buy In Option

Medicaid/CHIP buy-in programs for children with disabilities are being implemented in some states. This option allows states to expand Medicaid eligibility to children who meet certain disability and income criteria. This allows them to access Medicaid as either their only source of coverage, or in addition to private insurance, so they can access wrap-around additional coverage for their deductibles, co-pays and other uncovered health care costs.

Medicaid Waivers

Not all states offer TEFRA. However, as an alternative, many states have created Home and Community Based (HCBS) Waiver programs which provide expanded Medicaid coverage to children in higher income families who have developmental disabilities and/or significant medical needs. These programs are based solely on the child's need and not on the family's income. These waivers also allow states to target specific diagnoses or conditions. Medicaid waivers may provide personal care services, in-home or institutional respite, case management, home and vehicle modifications, nursing and palliative care, caregiver training and education, incontinence supplies, durable medical equipment, and assistive technology. Though these waivers can provide a tremendous amount of support to families, many states have limits/caps to the number of enrollees and therefore have extensive waiting lists. It is important that you take the time to sign up for these waivers early because of the length of time they take to get.

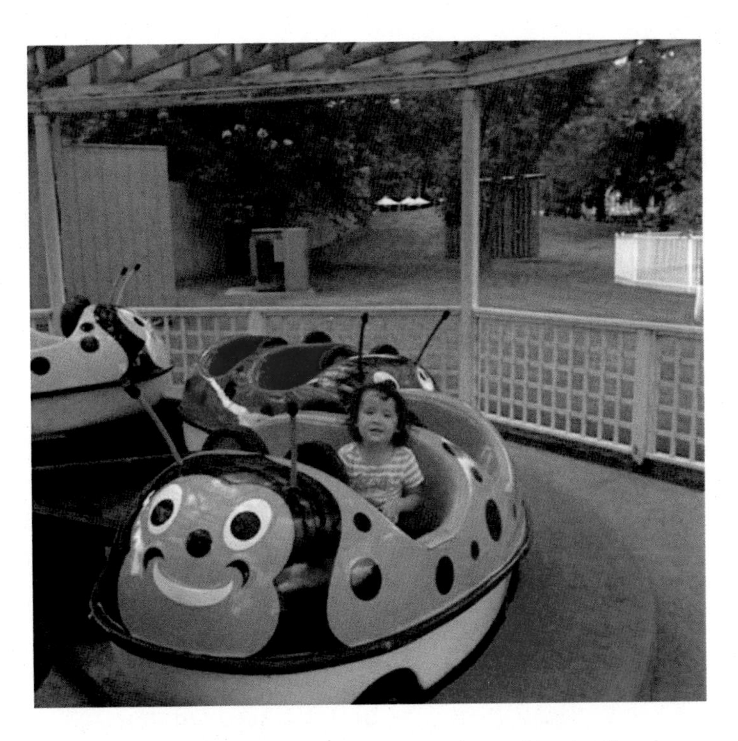

See the attached link for a State-by-State listing of Medicaid Waiver programs, http://www.medicaid.gov/medicaid-chip-program-information/by-topics/waivers/waivers_faceted.html or http://medicaidwaiver.org

Child-Only Insurance Policies

Child-only private insurance is defined as a class of coverage for an individual child who is less than 21 years old and has no spouse or dependents enrolled on the insurance contract. Parents often assume they have to enroll their child as a dependent on their group or independent health insurance, however child-only health policies may offer more flexibility with coverage (i.e which doctors you can see). It may be worth comparing their price and benefits as an alternative to enrolling a child as a dependent, or, in addition to group or family health plans.

Health Insurance Tips

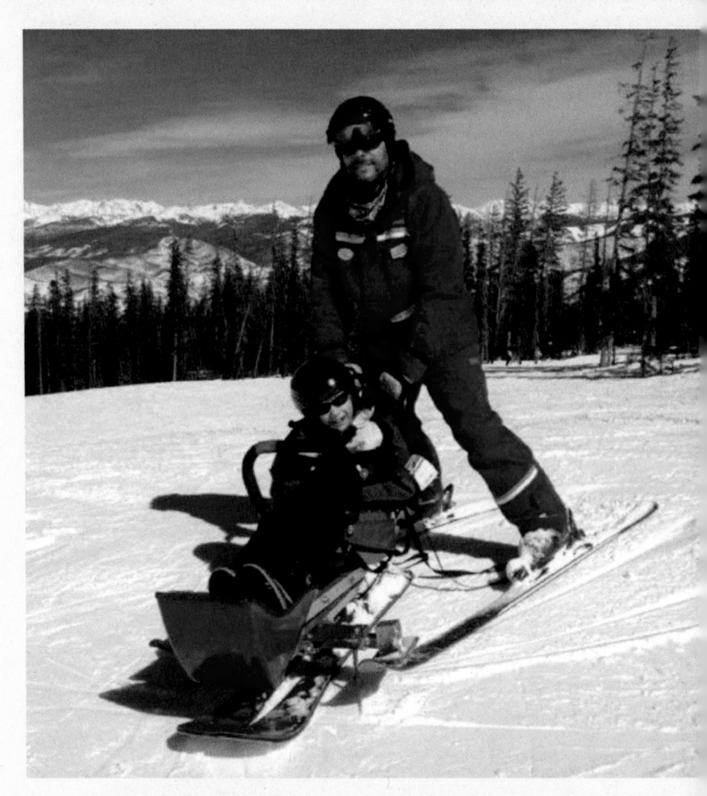

1. Talk to an insurance broker before purchasing any policy through the exchanges or private plans. You should not have to pay for the broker's services, (they earn credit or a percentage from the insurance carrier) and the broker can answer questions you may have about the specific needs of your child. For example, if your child is on a very expensive epilepsy drug, the broker can contact the insurance companies directly to determine how that will be covered. The same is true for specific therapies and equipment.

2. When deciding which type of policy to purchase, it may be beneficial to choose higher premiums that may have lower deductibles to avoid some higher out-of-pocket costs each year.

3. When deciding which type of policy to purchase, please consider that many families with children with CP have quite a few specialist visits, therapies, equipment and durable medical equipment. The more comprehensive "platinum" policies, though more expensive to purchase, may save you money in the long run.

4. Read your health insurance policy and take the time to familiarize yourself with your benefits and services. Some equipment and services will need prior authorization, prescriptions and letters of medical necessity, all of which are time-consuming and can be costly if the steps required by your insurance provider are not followed. By taking the time on the front end to familiarize yourself and to communicate with providers prior to receiv ing services or purchasing equipment, you can save crucial time and money.

5. Create a binder to save all Explanation of Benefits (EOB) from your insurance company.

6. Match bills from providers with their respective EOB's to make sure that they were processed correctly, that you are not being over-billed and that the insurance company is paying.

7. Health Care expenses are usually tax deductible. Save receipts, bills with the matching receipts of cancelled checks for tax purposes.

8. Medical travel may also be tax deductible, as well as expenses incurred by attending conferences or educational seminars related to your child's needs.

9. Health Insurance Premiums are often tax deductible for individuals who are self-employed.

10. Research TEFRA and Medicaid Waivers for your state and get on the waiting list.

11. TEFRA and Waivers should be in addition to your private or group policies if at all possible.

Achieving a Better Life Experience (ABLE) Act

The federal passage of the ABLE Act in 2014 amended the IRS tax code allowing states to establish tax-exempt savings programs for people with medically confirmed disabilities. The ABLE Act allows individuals with disabilities to save up to $100,000, on a tax-free basis, without jeopardizing their eligibility for Social Security or other benefits. States must pass their own bills to establish ABLE programs for their residents. These accounts are established and maintained by each state and managed by a financial institution, similar to a 529 college savings plan.

The purpose of the savings account is to support the health, independence and quality of life of the individual with a disability. Funds from the ABLE account can pay for education expenses, housing, transportation, employment training, assistive technology, personal care and support services, healthcare and more. It provides secure funding for disability-related expenses of beneficiaries with disabilities that will supplement, but not replace, benefits provided through private insurance, Supplemental Social Security Income, Medicaid, and other public benefits.

Special Needs Trusts

Your family may want to take advantage of setting up a Special Needs Trust (SNT). There are different reasons for wanting to set up a Special Needs Trust, but the main goal of such a trust is to provide for an individual with disabilities in a manner which does not adversely affect their qualification for benefits such as: Supplemental Security Income (SSI), Medical Assistance or Medicaid, and housing subsidies. The trust is structured such that the funds held by the trust supplement, rather than replace, government benefits. Unlike the ABLE Savings Accounts, a Special Needs Trust does not have a limit on the amount of funds that can be saved.

Some of the things that can be paid for by the funds in a Special Needs Trust are medical services and equipment not covered by government programs, computer devices and electronic equipment, recreational and cultural experiences, and furnishings, fitness equipment, and therapies not covered by government programs, among other things. Should an individual spend money from a Special Needs Trust on goods and services that otherwise would be provided through government programs such as Medicaid and SSI, they will be disqualified from the (government) program.

Because of the unique nature of these trusts, and the special requirements involved, it is recommended that, if possible, you consult with an attorney that practices in the area of Special Needs Law.

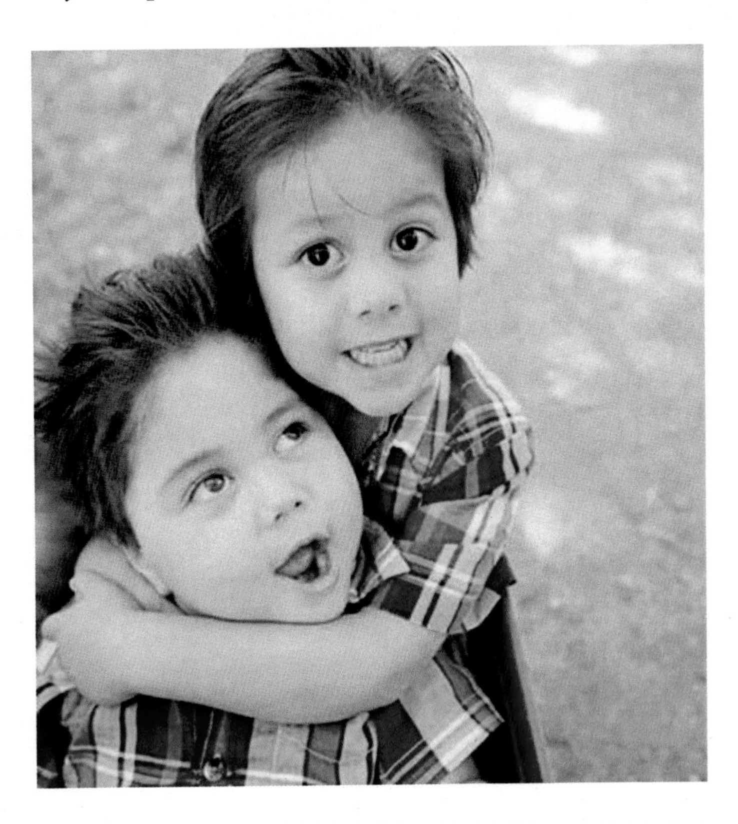

SECTION 11

Advocacy & Awareness Days

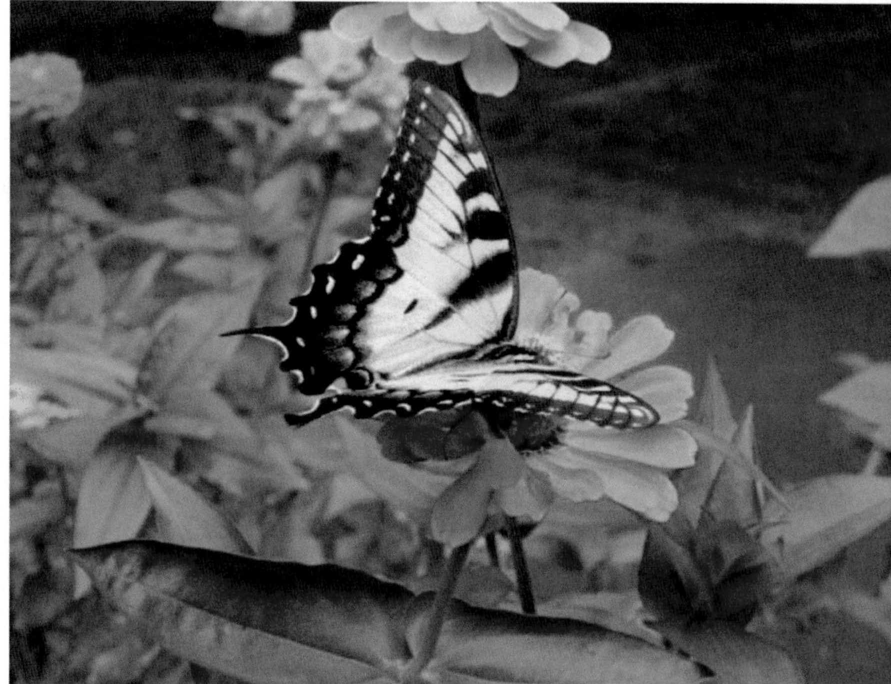

U.S. Cerebral Palsy Awareness Day

March 25

World CP Day

October 7
worldcpday.org

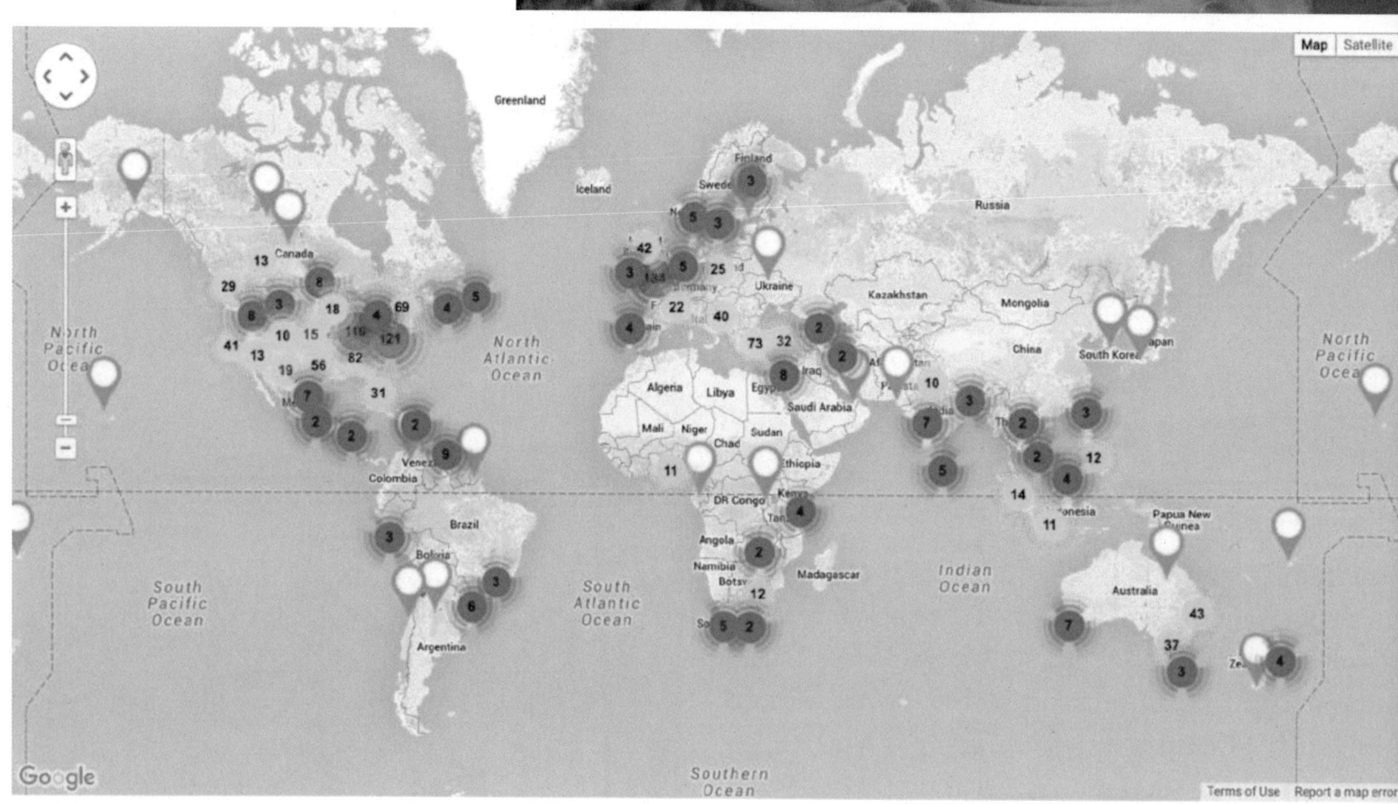

SECTION 12

Supportive Words from Other Parents

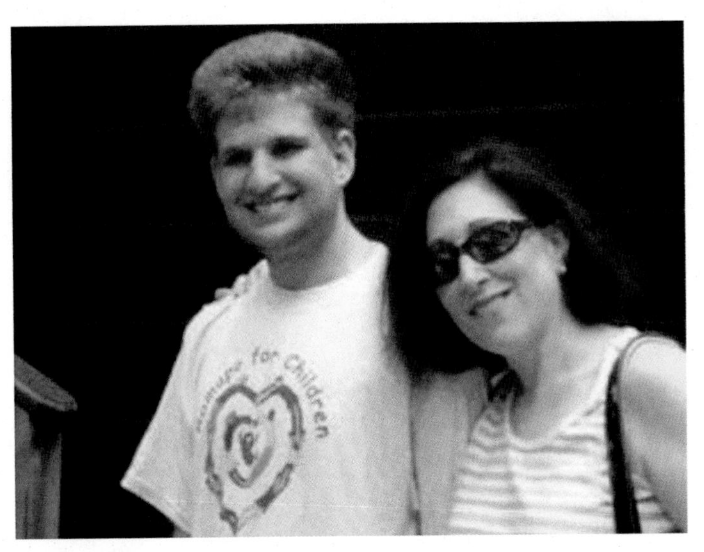

Liane Kupferberg Carter, author of *Ketchup is my Favorite Vegetable: A Family Grows Up With Autism*, wrote a very insightful for parents who have children with special needs called, "10 Things I Wish Someone Told Me About Parenting a Child with Special Needs." It was first published in Kveller magazine as well as the Huffington Post.

Courtesy of Ellen Seidman

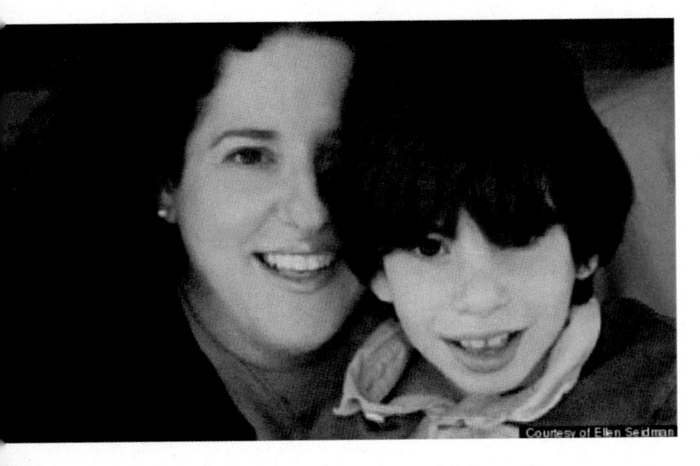

"What I Know About Motherhood Now that My Child Has Special Needs" was written by Ellen Seidman for the Huffington Post.

Mike
Father of two, one with cerebral palsy

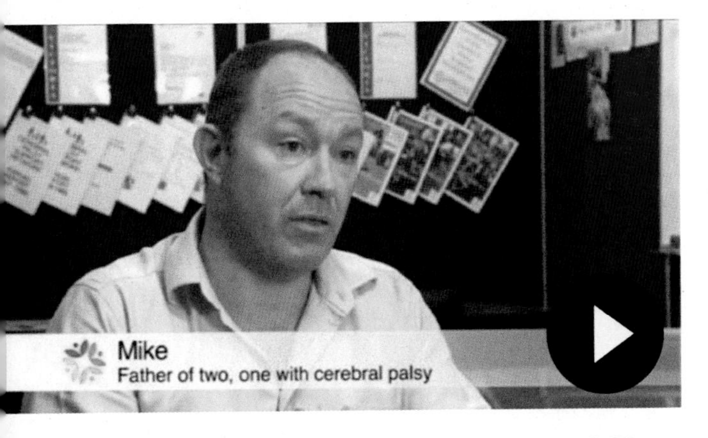

Here is a video about receiving a diagnosis of CP that was produced in Australia. It offers professional and parental perspectives. It is sourced from the "Raising Children website, 'Australia's trusted parenting website.'" For more parenting information, visit www.raisingchildren.net.au.

"Dear Mom of a Typical Kid": Are you feeling awkward around other mom's at the playground? Check out this beautifully written blog post from Dana Nieder who blogs at *Uncommon Sense*. She talks about her feelings and experience surrounding this issue. Her daughter Maya was five at the time the article was written, and she does not have a specific diagnosis.

SECTION 13

Additional Resources

CP Data and Statistics

Read the 2013 Cerebral Palsy Community Report put together by the US Centers for Disease Control and Prevention (CDC).

Local resources

Family Voices offers a directory of organizations by state that offer information to families. They include links to local disability resources centers and local parent to parent networks—i.e. parents of children with CP supporting other parents whose children also have CP: http://www.familyvoices.org/states

Below is The United Way's main website which offers access to countless resources and local organizations that may be helpful for you, your child and family. When you click on the link enter your zip code on the top right side. http://liveunited.org/. United Way also hosts a nationwide free, confidential, local human services information and referral service. For more information visit: http://211us.org/

AACPDM Professional Member Directory

American Academy for Cerebral Palsy and Developmental Medicine (AACPDM) provides a Professional Directory searchable by region to locate AACPDM professional members. *Please note that this directory is intended as a resource for locating a diversity of professionals who may be near you. The individuals included in the directory are not being specifically endorsed by CP NOW.

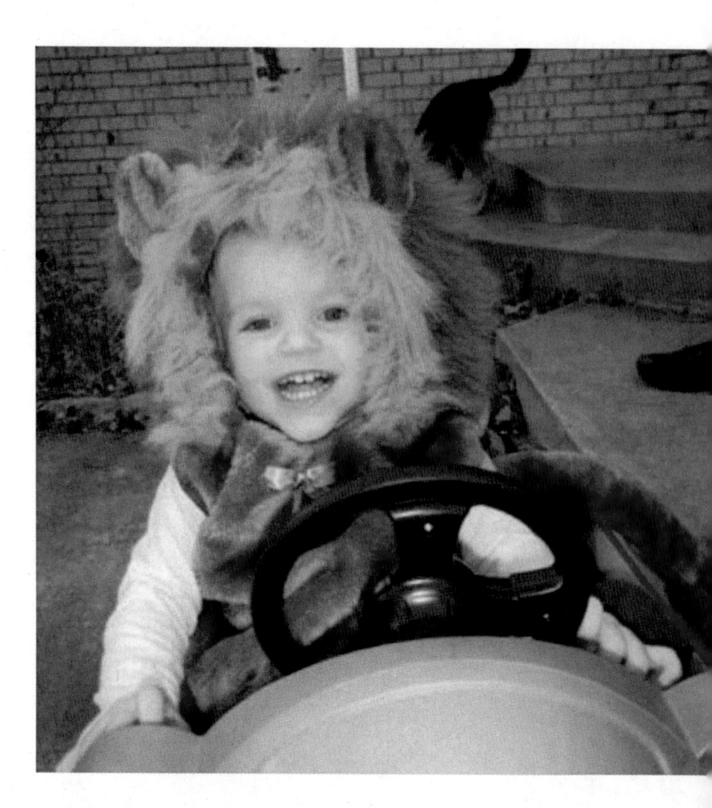

Assistive Technology

Closing the Gap—http://www.closingthegap.com is an excellent resource covering the latest assistive technology news, how to's and ever-changing technologies and implementation strategies.

General Child Care Resources and Information

→ Head Start
→ National Association for the Education of Young Children (NAEYC) Accredited Facility Search
→ Nationwide Easter Seals Directory of Child Development Centers
→ Inclusive Schools Network
→ From Early Intervention to Preschool: Information on Transitioning
→ States Without Preschool Education Programs

Useful links for finding facilities:

- Tips for Interviewing Daycare Facilities
- Tips For Parents of Special Needs Children Seeking Daycare

Insurance/Financial Planning Resources

The Catalyst Center is dedicated to improving health care coverage and financing for children and youth with special healthcare needs.

Possibilities — A financial resource website for parents of children with disabilities.

Preparing a Letter of Intent during the estate planning process: "The Letter of Intent", which is a not a legal document is the most important document that you can prepare in the estate planning process because it will help the people that will be caring for your child interpret your hopes and desires for your child." — from Friendship Circle of Michigan

Oral Health

The National Institute of Dental and Craniofacial Research

Respite Care

Lifespan Respite Care Act of 2006

Nationwide respite care search

Care.com — An international website that connects families with caregivers and caregiving companies.

Vision

(particularly resources for CVI)

American Foundation for the Blind (AFB)

North American Neuro-Ophthalmology Society

The Perkins School for the Blind offers excellent information and resources about CVI including many educational videos.

Books

General Reference

- *Cerebral Palsy: From Diagnosis to Adult Life*, Peter Rosenbaum and Lewis Rosenbloom
- *Cerebral Palsy: A Complete Guide for Caregiving*, Freeman Miller and Steven J. Bachrach
- *Children with Cerebral Palsy: A Parent's Guide*, Elaine Geralis
- *Finnie's Handling the Young Child with Cerebral Palsy*, Eva Bower, Editor

For Children

- *Ballerina Dreams*, Lauren Thompson
- *A Rainbow of Friends*, P.K. Hallinan
- *Rolling Along: The Story of Taylor and His Wheelchair*, Jamee Riggio Heelan

For Couples

- *Married with Special-Needs Children: A Couples' Guide to Keeping Connected*, Laura Marshak and Fran Prezant

For Dads

- *Uncommon Fathers: Reflections on Raising a Child with a Disability*, Donald J. Meyer

For Siblings

- *Views from Our Shoes: Growing Up with a Brother or Sister with Special Needs*, Donald J. Meyer

Insurance Reimbursement and Finances

- *The Special Needs Planning Guide*, John Nadworny CFP (Author), Cynthia Haddad CFP (Author)

SECTION 14

Contributors

Parent Contributors

Allison Combs
Alicia Champine
Lizette Dunay, Co-founder of Cure CP
Jennifer Lyman
Cheryl Major
Anna Meenan
Lori Poliski
Claire Paige-Reinhart
James Spinner
Blake Shusterman, MD
Michele Shusterman, Founder of CP Daily Living and CP NOW
Christina Youngblood

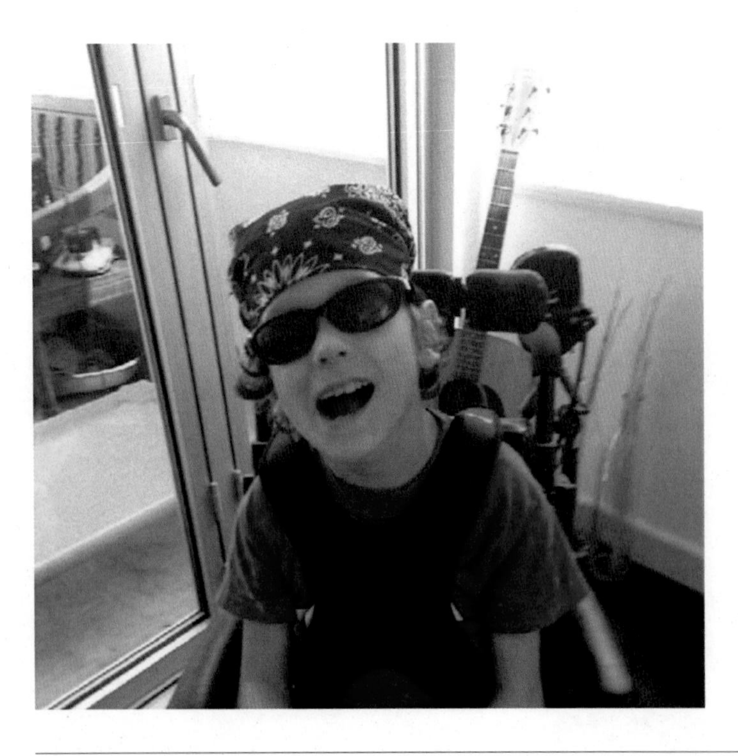

Adult Contributors (who have CP)

Dartania Emery
Ralph Strzalkowski Esquire
Emily W.
Julius Van der Wat
Steven Wampler
Kathleen Friel PhD

Professional Contributors & Reviewers

Meher Banajee, PhD, CCP-SLP, LSU Health Sciences Center Speech-Language Clinic.

Joseph Dutkowsky MD, Orthopedics, Associate Director, The Weinberg Family CP Center, Columbia University.

Heather Herdt OTR, Easter Seals, South Carolina.

Michael Kruer, MD, Screening section on **"Genetics"**—Neurology, Phoenix Children's Hospital.

Robert Mclaren MD, Urology, Mayo Clinic, Rochester, Minnesota.

Freeman Miller MD, **"Hip Surveillance"**—Orthopedics, Co-director of the CP and Medical Director of the Gait Analysis Laboratory at the AI duPont Institute.

Leah Morabito Esquire, **"Special Needs Trusts"**—Partner at Gimmel, Weiman, Ersek, Bloomberg & Lewis, P.A., Bethesda, MD.

Unni Narayanan, MD, MSc, FRCSC—Pediatric Orthopedic Surgery, The Hospital for Sick Children, Toronto, CA.

Ginny Paleg, PT, MPT, DScPT, Pediatric Physical Therapy, Types of therapy section—**"Physical Therapy."**

Wendy Pierce, MD, Pediatric Rehabilitation Medicine, Assistant Professor University of Colorado, Children's Hospital Colorado.

Christine Roman-Lantzy PhD, Screening section on **"Vision"**—Co-Director of Pediatric View in Pittsburgh, Pennsylvania.

Peter Rosenbaum MD, Developmental Pediatrics, Co-Founder of CanChild Center for Disability Research, Professor of Pediatrics McMaster University, Executive Director of CPnet.

Adrian Sandler MD, **"Coordinating Care"**—Developmental-Behavioral Pediatrics, Medical Director of Mission Hospital's Olson Huff Center for Child Development.

Richard Stevenson, MD, Screening section on **"Growth and Nutrition,"** Chief of Developmental & Behavioral Pediatrics, University of Virginia.

Lisa Thornton, MD, Pediatric Rehabilitation Physician and Medical Director of Pediatric and Adolescent Rehabilitation for Kids Rehab, a joint program between Schwab Rehabilitation Hospital and LaRabida Children's Hospital in Chicago. She is also assistant clinical professor in the departments of Pediatrics, and Orthopedics & Rehabilitation at the University of Chicago Pritzker School of Medicine.

Andy Zabel, PhD, **"Neuropsychology Assessments"**—Clinical Director Neuropsychology, Kennedy Krieger Institute, Baltimore, Maryland.

Special Thanks

The Occupational Therapy team and Andrea Hauck Photograpy of the Meyer Center for Special Children

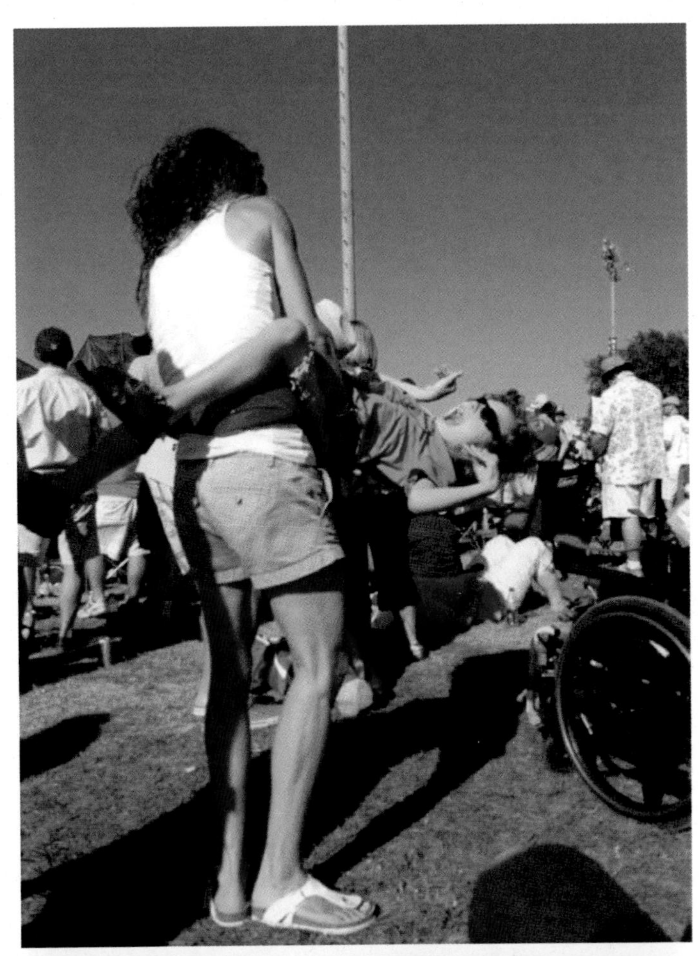

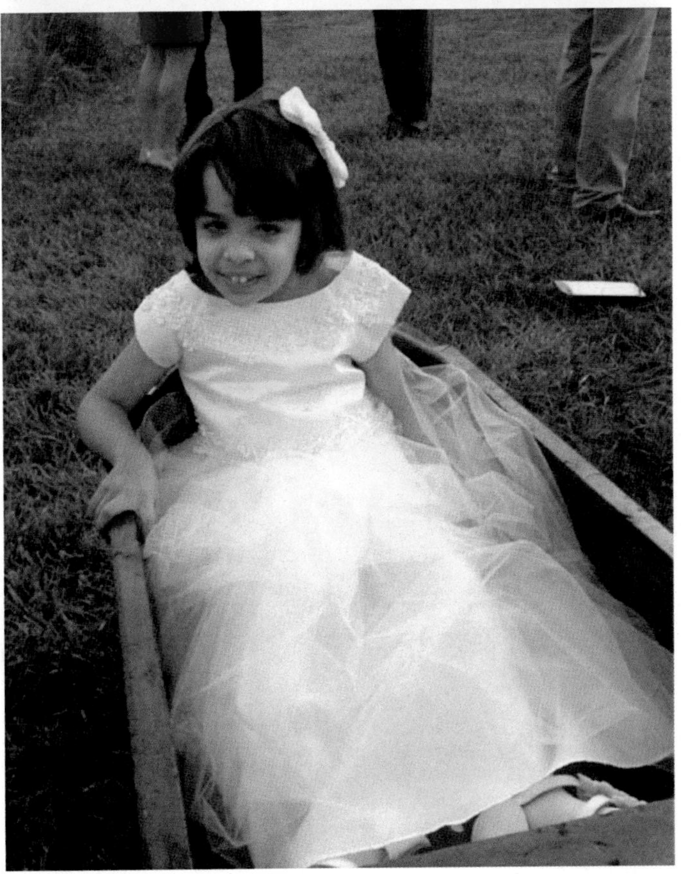

SECTION 15

References

1. Surveillance of Cerebral Palsy in Europe (SCPE). Surveillance of cerebral palsy in Europe: a collaboration of cerebral palsy surveys and registers. *Dev Med Child Neurol*. 2000; 42(12):816-24.
2. Christensen D, Van Naarden Braun K, Doernberg NS et al. Prevalence of cerebral palsy, co-occurring autism spectrum disorders, and motor functioning. *Dev Med Child Neurol*. 2014; 56(1):59-65.
3. Movement Disorder Society. Definition and Classifications of Hyperkinetic Movements in Childhood. *Movement Disorders* 2010;25 (11): 1538–1549.
4. Movement Disorder Society, 1542-1543.
5. Morris JG, Jankelowitz SK, Fung VS, Clouston PD, et al. Athetosis I: historical considerations. *Movement Disorders* 2002; 17;1278-1280
6. Movement Disorder Society, 1542.
7. Blackman J. UCP's Medical Directors' Desk. Family Centered Care. http://ucp.org/resources/from-the-medical-director-s-desk/family-centered-care/ Accessed November 15, 2015.
8. King S, Teplicky R, King G, et al. Family-centered service for children with cerebral palsy and their families: A review of the literature. *Seminars in Pediatric Neurology* 2004;11: 78-86.
9. National Institutes of Health (NIH). NIH Fact Sheets-Newborn Hearing Screening. http://report.nih.gov/NIHfactsheets/ViewFactSheet.aspx?csid=104 Accessed November 15, 2015.
10. Reid SM1, Modak MB, Berkowitz RG et al. A population-based study and systematic review of hearing loss in children with cerebral palsy. *Dev Med Child Neurol*. 2011 53(11):1038-45.
11. Penner M, Xie W, Binepal N et al. Characteristics of pain in youth and children with cerebral palsy. *Pediatrics*; originally published online July 15, 2013; DOI: 10.1542/peds.2013-0224.
12. Paris B, Murray-Slutsky C. Star Services. Integrating Neurodevelopmental Treatment and Sensory Integration-Theory and Practice in the Client with Cerebral Palsy. http://www.starservices.tv/images/Integrating_NDT_and_SI-Theory_and_Practice-CMS.pdf Accessed November 15, 2015.
13. Council on Children with Disabilities (COCWD) of the American Academy of Pediatrics (AAP). Policy Statement: Sensory Integration Therapies for Children with Developmental and Behavioral Disorders. http://pediatrics.aappublications.org/content/129/6/1186.full. Published June 2012. Accessed November 15, 2015.
14. Penner, e407.
15. Cummings, S., Canadian Paediatric Society, & Community Paediatrics Committee. Melatonin for the management of sleep disorders in children and adolescents. *Paediatric Child Health*, 2012 17(6); 331-333.
16. Galland B. Elder D., and Taylor B. Interventions with a sleep outcome for children with cerebral palsy or a post-traumatic brain injury: A systematic review. *Sleep Medicine Reviews*. 2012;16: 561-573.
17. Mindell J, Kuhn B, Lewin, et al. Behavioral treatment of bedtime problems and night wakings in infants and young children. 2006; *Sleep*. 29(10): 1263-1276.
18. Weiss T. Sleep Issues and Children With Developmental Disorders. *Disabled World*. December 21, 2013. http://www.disabled-world.com/health/neurology/sleepdisorders/cdd.php. Accessed November 15, 2015.

9 Murphy K, Boutin S, Ride K. Cerebral palsy, neurogenic bladder, and outcomes of lifetime care. 2012 *Dev Med Child Neurol*. 54: 945-950.
20 Flanagan NM, Jackson AJ, Hill AE. Visual impairment in childhood: insights from a community-based survey. *Child Care Health Dev* 2003;29(6):493-9.
21 Good WV, Jan JE, DeSa L, Barkovich AJ, Groenveld M, Hoyt CS. Cortical visual impairment in children. *Surv Ophthalmol* 1994;38(4):351-64.
22 Steinkuller PG, Du L, Gilbert C, Foster A, Collins ML, Coats DK. Childhood blindness. *J Aapos* 1999;3(1):26-32.
23 Family Connection SC. An Unexpected Treasure. http://www.familyconnectionsc.org/uploads/1/7/2/7/17273542/an_unexpected_treasure.pdf Accessed November 15, 2015.
24 Rosenbaum P. (2015 March). CP-NET Webinar Series - Complementary and Alternative Therapy https://vimeo.com/120597054
25 Rosenbaum P. CP-NET Webinar Series-Complementary and Alternative Therapy.
26 Movement Disorder Society, 1540.

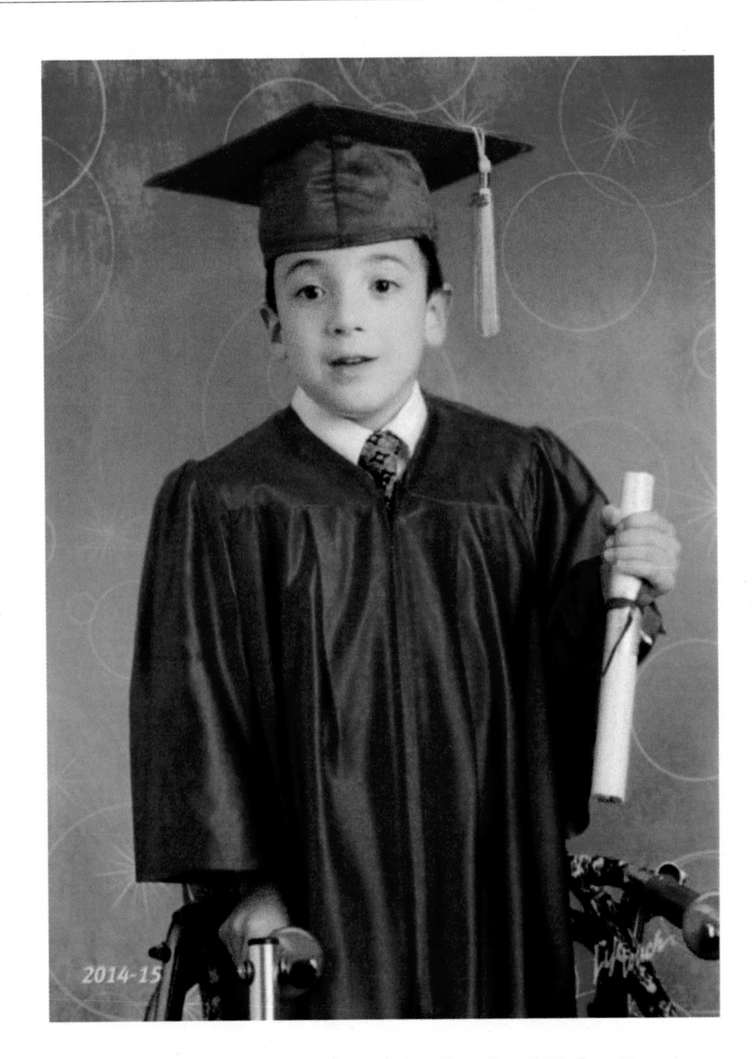

Additional Sources

Can CHILD. Keeping Current: Sleep Issues Among Children with Cerebral Palsy. http://cpnet.canchild.ca/en/resources/KeepingCurrentonSleep.pdf Accessed October 10, 2015.

Combs A. "Urinary Incontinence in CP". Lecture presented at The Weinberg Family CP Center educational conference for professionals, families and adults with CP; May 18, 2013. New York, NY.

Kuperminc M, Stevenson R. Growth and Nutrition Disorders in Children with Cerebral Palsy. 2008; *Dev Disabil* Res Rev. 14(2): 137-146.

NINDS Information on stem cell research. http://www.ninds.nih.gov/research/stem_cell/ Updated October, 20, 2015. Accessed November 15, 2015.

Rosenbaum P, Rosenbloom L. *Cerebral Palsy From Diagnosis to Adult Life*. London, England: Mac Keith Press; 2012

Surveillance of Cerebral Palsy in Europe. http://www.scpenetwork.eu/en/publications/scpe-collaboration/

Part of the sibling support section was written using NICHCY News Digest 20, 3rd Edition, 2003. NICCHY no longer exists and their material is not copyrighted but they request that their material be mentioned. http://www.parentcenterhub.org/nichcy-gone/

SECTION 16

Glossary

A

Abduction — The movement of a leg or arm away from the midline of the body.

Accessibility — The degree to which a product, device, service, or environment is available to as many people as possible.

Accommodations — Removing obstacles that impede accessibility, thereby helping a person with disabilities function and participate in a typical environment.

ADLs — Activities of daily living such as toileting and feeding.

Adaptive equipment — Physical props or supports to aid those with special needs. (i.e. corner chair, prone board, etc)

Adaptive Equipment Specialist/Vendor of Medical Equipment — Evaluates a patient's ability to use assistive technology devices; fits, fabricates or modifies equipment; and assesses equipment needs for home, work or school.

Adduction — Inward movement of a leg or arm toward the body.

Advocacy — Speaking on behalf of a person, cause, or group to support or promote their actions.

Alternative Medicine — Approaches to medical care and treatment used in place of standard medical practice. Also see Complementary and Alternative Medicines (CAMs)

Amblyopia — (also known as 'lazy eye') — the loss or lack of development of central vision in one eye.

Ambulatory — The ability to walk.

Americans with Disabilities Act (ADA) — A federal law that prohibits discrimination of the disabled by employers, public accommodations, public and private services, and in telecommunications. Failure to make reasonable accommodations is considered discrimination.

Ankle foot orthosis (AFO) — A type of brace surrounding the ankle and at least part of the foot that is used to support proper positioning in these areas.

Articulation — The ability to move and control all parts of the mouth to make the sounds of a language.

Aspirate — To suck or draw in food or liquids into the lungs by inhaling. Children with CP may swallow improperly while drinking and get a small portion in their lungs.

Assessment (or evaluation) — Process to determine a child's strengths and weaknesses; includes testing and observations performed by a team of specialists.

Assistive technology (AT) — Any item, piece of equipment, or product system used to increase, maintain, or improve the functional capabilities of a child with a disability.

ATA-Assistive Technology Act — An act which seeks to provide assistive technology to persons with disabilities so they can more fully participate in education, employment, and daily activities on a level playing field with other members of their communities.

Assistive Technology Professional (ATP) — An ATP is an individual who is has demonstrated competence (through RESNA) in analyzing the needs of consumers with disabilities, assisting in the selection of appropriate assistive technology for the consumer's needs, and providing training in the use of the selected device(s).

Astigmatism — Blurry vision due to either the irregular shape of the cornea, the clear front cover of the eye, or sometimes the curvature of the lens inside the eye.

Asymmetrical — When one side of the body is different from the other.

Atrophy — To deteriorate or progressively weaken. Refers to muscle tissue in children with CP.

Audiologist — Provides customized hearing assessments and diagnostic testing.

Auditory processing — Being able to understand individual speech sounds quickly enough to comprehend the meaning of what is being spoken.

B

Basal ganglia — a group of structures in the base of the brain involved in movement and coordination.

Brain plasticity — See Neuroplasticity.

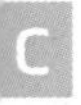

Case manager — Person responsible for coordinating services and information from a multidisciplinary team.

Central nervous system — The brain and spinal cord. Mainly controls voluntary movement and thought processes.

Cerebellum — Part of the brain that helps coordinate muscle activity and control balance.

Cerebral palsy — Movement and posture disorder resulting from non-progressive damage to the developing brain.

Cerebrospinal fluid — A clear liquid that constantly surrounds the spinal cord and flows through the ventricles of the brain. It acts as a protective cushion and nourishes the areas it surrounds.

Child life specialist — Helps children cope with hospitalization and medical procedures through therapeutic play and child-appropriate hospital tours. Specialists also meet with siblings (to address their questions and concerns) and involve patients and siblings in activities.

Child development — A process of learning and mastering skills in the areas of gross, fine motor, speech and language development, social and emotional development and cognitive development. Choreoathetosis — A type of CP that results in a variety of muscle tone and involuntary movements of the limbs.

Constraint Induced Movement Therapy (CIMT) — CIMT plus Bimanual Training (BIT) is a type of therapy directed by an occupational therapist for individuals who have difficulty using one arm or hand. They often have decreased range of motion, strength, coordination and sensation in one of their upper extremities which often affects their ability to complete activities that require the use of two hands. CIMT limits use of the better arm by wearing a constraint and provides intensive practice for the weaker arm.

Clinical trial — A clinical study involves research using human volunteers (also called participants) that is intended to add to medical knowledge.

Clonus — Fast alternating relaxation and contraction of the muscles caused by spastic muscles.

Cognition — The ability to process and understand the surrounding environment. (thinking)

Combat crawling — Crawling while on stomach and using mostly your arms to pull the rest of the body forward.

Complementary and alternative medicines (CAMS) — Complementary and alternative medicine (CAMS) is a term for medical products and practices that are not part of standard medical care/practice. Complementary medicine is used together with standard medical treatment with the goal of supporting or enhancing its effects, or alleviating its side effects. Alternative medicine is used in place of standard medical practices or approaches to treatment.[25]

Congenital — A condition present at birth.

Cortical visual impairment (CVI) — A neurological condition that is the leading cause of visual impairment of children in the US and the First World and is commonly seen in people with cerebral palsy. It is not an eye condition.

CT scan (computerized axial tomography) — A medical imaging technique that produces multiple images of the inside of the body

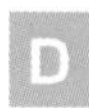

Development — See Child development.

Developmental delay — Any delay in physical, cognitive (processing info/thinking), social, emotional, communication, or adaptive (self-help skills) development. It is typically used as a label under IDEA to qualify children between 3-9 for special education service. The percentage of delay to qualify for these services varies from state to state.

Developmental disability — A condition causing an impairment in learning, language, or behavior areas. About one in six children in the U.S. have one or more developmental disabilities or other developmental delays (source CDC).

Developmental milestone — A developmental goal, such as sitting or using two-word phrases, which health care providers use to measure developmental progress over time.

Developmental pediatrician — A pediatrician who specializes in developmental milestones and assessing normal or abnormal child development.

Differentiation — A discrimination between things as different and distinct.

Diplegia — A term used in CP (typically the spastic form) that refers to mobility or muscle tone abnormalities affecting an individual's legs.

Durable Medical Equipment (DME) — Supportive medical equipment used to improve the quality of life and independence of the user. Examples include wheelchairs, bathing chairs, standers etc.

DNA — Short for deoxyribonucleic acid, which is a complex molecule that contains all of the information necessary to build and maintain an organism.

Dysphagia — Difficulty swallowing.

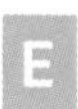

Early intervention — Therapy and family instruction provided for children ages birth to three years old that is intended to minimize presentation of developmental delay.

Early interventionist (EI) — A person who arranges for a therapist to come to the house or meet at the family at a facility for treatment and provides family training to have the family incorporate practical ideas to improve child's development in-between therapy sessions.

EEG-Electroencephalogram — A test that charts the level of electrical discharge from nerve cells in the brain. It is used to test for abnormal brain/seizure activity.

Epilepsy — A neurological disorder in which nerve cells in the brain have unusual activity causing a person's consciousness, movement, or actions may be altered for a short time.

Equilibrium — A child's sense or actual physical balance.

:quinus — Walking on toes because the calf nuscles are shortened or contracted.

:xpressive language — Verbal, written, or use of ;estures to communicate.

:xtension — Straightening the limbs or trunk.

:xtrapyramidal — The movement disorders ncluded in dyskinetic CP (chorea, dystonia and ıthetosis) are among the hyperkinetic (unwanted, ›xcess movement) motor abnormalities associated vith the concept of "extrapyramidal" in adults. The term has sometimes been used by clinicians to lescribe types of CP. However, in 2008 the Task-'orce on Childhood Movement Disorders met at the National Institutes of Health and agreed that this erm lacks accuracy and they recommended not ısing it to describe movement disorders in chil-lren.[26]

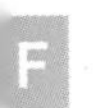

Feeding tube — A tube of soft plastic used in feed-ing for those who have difficulty getting enough nutrition through regular eating. (29)

Femoral bone (femur) — Thigh bone.

Femoral torsion (femoral anteversion) — Inward twisting of the femur so that the knees and feet turn inward.

Fine motor skills — Using small muscle groups, such as face, hands, feet, fingers, toes. Fine motor skills include feeding, holding an object between thumb and fore finger (pincer grasp), turning/twisting, etc.

Flexion — Bending of joints.

Flexor — A muscle controlling the bending of joints.

Floppy — Loose movements and weak posture.

Fluctuating tone — Combination of loose and tight muscles in different areas.

Focal motor seizures — Jerking of a few muscles without an immediate loss of consciousness.

Foot drop (drop foot) — Gait abnormality charac-terized by trouble lifting the front part of the foot.

Functional vision — Refers to how an individual uses his/her vision in everyday life.

Gag reflex — A reflex that can often be extra sensi-tive with those with cerebral palsy, to the point where the child may gag or choke when something touches their tongue or palate. Over sensitization of the oral reflexes are often addressed by occupa-tional therapist, speech language pathologist, or physical therapist.

Gait — The way (or manner) in which someone walks.

Gait analysis — The study of how a someone walks.

Gait trainer — A device that acts like a walker but with supports to stabilize the hips and ankles to encourage good posture and placement of feet and legs while walking.

Gastroesophageal reflux (GERD) — A digestive disease in which the stomach acid flows back into the esophagus.

Gastrostomy tube — G-Tube is a tube inserted through the abdomen that delivers nutrition directly to the stomach.

General movements (GMs) — Body movement present from early fetal life onwards until and after birth (up to 18 weeks post-term). They involve the whole body in a variable sequence of arm, leg, neck, and trunk movements. They change in intensity, force and speed, and they have a gradual beginning and end. If the nervous system is impaired, GMs loose their complex and variable character and become monotonous.

General Movements Assessment — A quick, non-invasive and cost-effective way to identify neurological issues which may lead to cerebral palsy and other developmental disabilities. The assessment can be conducted from birth to 3 months of age by analyzing the child's GMs. The GMA was developed by Professor Heinz Prechtl, a Developmental Neurologist, from Graz in Austria.

GMFCS (Gross Motor Function Classification System) — A 5-level classification system that describes the gross motor function of children and youth with cerebral palsy. It's intended to replace the very subjective terms of "mild", "moderate", and "severe".

Gross motor — Using large muscle groups, such as legs, arms, and abdomen. Gross motor skills include transitioning between postures, standing, walking, running, jumping, etc.

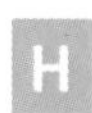

Head control — The ability to control movement of the head.

Hemiplegia — A type of cerebral palsy that refers to either the right or the left side of the body being affected by abnormal muscle tone, movement, and/ or control.

High tone — Tightness, or spasticity, of the muscles.

Hip dislocation — Occurs when the ball shaped end of the femur comes out of its socket in the pelvis.

Hip subluxation — See Subluxation.

Hydrocephalus — A blockage of the flow of cerebrospinal fluid that increases pressure in the ventricles of the brain. Can cause brain damage. Often relieved by surgical insertion of a tube called a shunt to drain the fluid.

Hypertonia — Increased tension in the muscles, also known as high tone.

Hypotonia — Decreased tension in the muscles, also known as low tone.

Impairment — Decrease in strength, dexterity or ability to use a leg, arm or other body part.

IFSP (Individualized Family Service Plan) — Pertains to children three and younger. Usually set up by an early interventionist (EI). The family and the EI discuss areas of development that the child needs improvement on, set goals, and lists different methods to work on improving those areas. It is updated at least every six months.

Inclusion — Being included or involved in a typical classroom as much as the child's disability will allow (see also least restrictive environment under IDEA).

Incontinence — lack of control of bladder or bowel movements.

Inhibition — Movements and positioning which discourage muscle tightness.

Input — Information received through any of the five senses that can be used to learn new skills.

Intellectual Disability — A child who, before eighteen, has below average intellectual functioning and self-help behavior.

Interdisciplinary team — A team of professionals from varying fields (teacher, therapists, doctors) who evaluate a child and then develop a summary of the child's abilities, progress, and needs in each of their areas of expertise to get a total picture of each area of the child's life.

Intracerebral — Within the brain.

Intracranial — Within the skull.

n utero — Literally in the uterus, referring to the eriod of time during fetal development.

nversion — When a part of the body turns in.

nvoluntary movements — uncontrolled movenents.

K

nee ankle foot orthosis (KAFO) — A long lastic leg brace, which supports the whole leg, and inges at the knee.

earning disability — A child with normal inteligence who has difficulty processing certain types f information.

Lesion — An area of abnormal tissue change

Long-leg sitting — Sitting with legs extended in ront of the body.

Low tone — Decreased muscle tone.

Lower extremities — Legs.

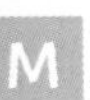

Manual Ability Classification System (MACS) — Describes how children with cerebral palsy use their hands to manipulate objects.

Magnetic resonance imaging (MRI) scan — Medical technique used to see the details of structures inside the body.

Medicaid — A state and federal program that offers medical assistance for those eligible to receive Supplementary Security Income (SSI). TEFRA programs are a form of Medicaid (not available in all states) but the income criteria is based on the child's resources rather than the entire family.

Midline — An imaginary reference line separating the right side of the body from the left. Most often used in doctor's and therapy notes.

Motor — Ability to move oneself.

Motor delay — Slower development of movement skills.

Motor patterns — Ways in which the body and limbs work together to make sequenced movement.

Motor planning — The ability to think through and carry out a physical task

Muscle tone — The amount of resistance or tension during rest or in response to stretching

Neurodevelopmental pediatrician — Provides consultations for the evaluation and diagnosis of children with neurological developmental disabilities.

Neurologist — A physician who specializes in disorders of the nervous system.

Neuromotor — Involving the nerves and muscles.

Neuroplasticity — The brain's ability to reorganize and change itself by forming new connections.

Neuropsychologist — Helps assess and treat developmental, medical, psychiatric, and neurological conditions or problems; might work with developmental pediatricians, pediatric neurologists, child psychiatrists, pediatricians, occupational therapists, and speech and language therapists.

Nissen fundoplication — A surgical procedure used to treat Gastroesophageal Reflux (GERD) and Hiatal Hernias. It is used to treat GERD when all other interventions have failed. The procedure involves wrapping the upper end of the stomach around the lower end of the esophagus and then stitched into place therefore reinforcing the closing ability of the esophageal sphincter.

O

"Off label" prescription — Refers to the use of a medication outside the specifications outlined in the FDA's approved medication packaging label, or insert. "Off-label" prescribing is legal and very common. Off label use of drugs can be beneficial, especially when patients have exhausted all other proven options. However, it is important to discuss potential risks/benefits with your medical team. This link offers additional information about off-label prescriptions. http://www.webmd.com/a-to-z-guides/features/off-label-drug-use-what-you-need-to-know

Oral motor — Control of lip, tongue and jaw muscles.

Orthopedic — Relating to the joints, ligaments, bones, and muscles.

Orthopedic disability — An impairment that affects the bones, muscles, or joints as well as the ability to perform in other developmental areas. This particular label can be used for children with cerebral palsy to get special education services.

Orthopedist vs. Podiatrist — An orthopedist is a doctor who specializes in preventing or correcting problems related to the joints, ligaments, bones and muscles, whereas a podiatrist is a doctor who specializes in preventing or correcting problems related to the feet.

Orthoses (Orthotics) — Lightweight devices that provide stability at the joints or passively stretch the muscles. Can be made of plastic, metal, or leather.

Orthotist — Designs, fabricates and fits a wide variety of orthoses (braces) for upper and lower limbs, the spine and the hips.

Osteotomy — An operation to cut and realign the bones. Ex: to change the angles of the femoral bone and the hip joint.

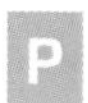

P

Parent advocate — A parent with knowledge and/or training about special education law and who provides advocacy support to fellow parents facing obstacles obtaining an education and related accommodations for his/her child.

Parent to parent organization — An organization staffed by parents who provide support and resources to other parents facing similar challenges raising their children.

Patching — See Eye patching.

Pediatric neurologist — Evaluates, diagnoses and treats neurological conditions. Pediatric neurologists manage seizures and collaborate with pediatric rehabilitation medicine physicians to recommend interventions for some associated conditions, such as learning, behavior and sensory issues.

Pediatric neurosurgeon — Provides comprehensive surgical care for patients who have medical conditions that affect the spine, neck, nerves and/or brain. A pediatric neurosurgeon might perform surgeries such as implant shunts to reduce excessive fluid pressure in the brain; or implant vagus nerve stimulators to reduce the occurrence of seizures; or intrathecal baclofen pump to reduce spasticity..

Pediatric orthopedist — Examines a patient's bones, muscle structure and joint movements in relation to posture, function and gait. An orthopedist might perform surgery to improve the function of a child's legs or arms as he or she grows.

Pediatric rehabilitation medicine physician — Specializes in rehabilitation services—including therapy, orthotics, and oral or injectable medicines—and recommends specialized equipment.

Perception — Perception is the making sense of information gained from the senses. This enables hildren to do things such as move around obsta-les, judge size and shape of objects and under-stand how lines are connected to form letters. For hose who experience problems with these, it may not become apparent until school or preschool.

Peripheral Nervous System — The part of the nervous system that consists of the nerves and ganglia outside of the brain and spinal cord.

Physical therapy — Evaluation and treatments aimed at helping people improve gross-motor skills, strength and balance. Therapists also recommend, create and customize adaptive equipment, such as power or manual wheelchairs, walkers, and standers.

Podiatrist — A doctor of podiatric medicine (DPM), diagnose and treat conditions of the foot, ankle, and related structures of the leg.

Posture — Positioning or alignment of the body

Pragmatics — Understanding how and why language is used.

Primitive reflexes — Early patterns of movement in a child that usually disappear after about six months of age.

Proprioception — Sensing or perceiving where one's body and its individual parts are in physical space

Psychologist — Evaluates patient's' cognitive, academic and psychosocial abilities. Psychologists talk with patients and families about the effects of a disability and help cope with pain and stress. May also contact patients' schools to discuss special academic services or behavior-management strategies.

Q

Quadriplegia — A term used to describe cases of cerebral palsy in which the entire body is affected.

R

Range of motion (ROM) — The degree of motion present at a joint.

Receptive language — The ability to understand what is written or being said.

Reflex — An involuntary movement in response to stimulation such as touch, pressure or joint movement.

Reinforcement — Providing a pleasant consequence (such as getting to do favorite activity or eat favorite food) or removing an unpleasant consequence (such as a chore or a punishment that was in place) after a behavior in order to increase or maintain that behavior.

Respite care — Publicly funded skilled care and supervision of a person with disabilities in the family's or caregiver's home. Usually available for several hours per week or for overnight stay.

Scissoring gait — Crossing of the legs together when walking.

Scoliosis — Curvature of the spine.

Seizure — Involuntary movement or changes in consciousness or behavior brought on by an abnormal burst of electrical activity in the brain.

Selective motor control — See Loss of Selective Motor Control.

Sensation — Loss of feeling (touch) may affect some children with cerebral palsy in their performance of both fine and gross motor tasks. This will depend on the degree of involvement of the limbs. This loss of feeling is often linked with a lack of awareness of their limbs and the child may need encouragement to use the limbs that are affected.

Sensory integration disorders — Disorders affecting the brain's ability to integrate information processed from the five senses.

Service coordinator — A professional who arranges services and referrals for a person with special needs. These services can be medical, therapeutic, educational, material goods or even social in nature. Most typically associated with early intervention but other organizations provide service coordination as well.

Shunt — A device used to drain excess spinal fluid from the brain for those with hydrocephalus.

Side sitting — Sitting with both knees bent and to one side of the body.

Spasticity — Abnormal, stiff muscle tone making movement difficult.

Special education — Specialized instruction based on educational disabilities determined by a team evaluation. It must be relevant to their educational needs and adapted to the child's learning style.

Special needs — Refers to the individual support required by an individual with disabilities

Special needs trust — A specialized legal document designed to benefit an individual who has a disability. Also referred to as a supplemental needs trust.

Speech and language pathology — Therapy to treat speech and language disorders including receptive language and expressive language.

Strabismus — A disorder where the eyes do not line up in the same direction.

Subluxation — Partial dislocation of any joint. Ex: when the head of the thigh bone (femur) moves out of its normally centered position in the hip socket.

Supramalleolar orthoses (SMO's) — A type of ankle-foot orthosis (AFO's) designed to support the leg above the ankle bones.

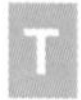

Tactile — Related to the sense of touch.

Toe walking — walking on toes without heel-strike.

Unilateral — One-sided.

Upper extremities — Arms.

Urodynamic testing — Any procedure that looks at how well the bladder, sphincters, and urethra are storing and releasing urine.

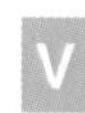

Vestibular system — Refers to vestibular system including the inner ear and areas of the brain that help control balance and eye movements.

VCUG or Voiding cystourethrogram — This diagnostic X-ray test helps to determine the bladder capacity and emptying ability and to detect abnormalities of the urethra and the bladder.

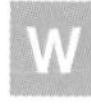

Weakness — Lacking muscle strength.

W-sitting — Sitting on your bottom with knee bent and feet pointed out to either side of the hips.

info@cpnowfoundation.org

COVER PHOTO https://www.flickr.com/photos/slgc

DESIGN KUDOS Design Collaboratory

Made in the USA
Monee, IL
17 May 2022